The
ersonalized
et

Eran Segal, PhD, and Eran Elinav, MD, PhD

WITH EVE ADAMSON

The **Personalized** Diet

Why One-Size-Fits-All Diets Don't Work

Vermilion
LONDON

1 3 5 7 9 10 8 6 4 2

Vermilion, an imprint of Ebury Publishing,
20 Vauxhall Bridge Road,
London SW1V 2SA

Vermilion is part of the Penguin Random House group of companies whose
addresses can be found at global.penguinrandomhouse.com

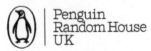

Penguin
Random House
UK

First published in the United Kingdom by Vermilion in 2017
First published in the United States by Grand Central Publishing in 2017
www.penguin.co.uk

A CIP catalogue record for this book is available from the British Library

ISBN 9781785041303

Printed and bound in Great Britain by Clays Ltd, St Ives PLC

Penguin Random House is committed to a sustainable future for our
business, our readers and our planet. This book is made from Forest
Stewardship Council® certified paper.

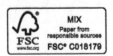

To our teachers, colleagues, and students for making our joint truth-pursuing journey an enjoyable and moving experience

CONTENTS

PART I
A Twenty-First-Century Epidemic and the Personalized Nutrition Solution

PART II
The Personalized Diet Program

ACKNOWLEDGMENTS

The Personalized Diet is a culmination of two years of extensive effort. It translates a large set of results and discoveries stemming from years of grueling scientific research performed at our two labs into a story that is easy to grasp for nonscientists and touches upon the very basis of our lives: our diet, health, risk of becoming obese and developing diabetes and many other "modern diseases," and the mysterious bacteria that live within us and with us and make us who we are.

We are grateful to our agent, Alex Glass, for recognizing that this story should be brought into the broad public and for initiating, assisting, and guiding us throughout the process. We are deeply indebted to Eve Adamson, who has spent countless hours brainstorming, writing, and editing with us, in an effort to bridge the gap between science and common knowledge, to make this book accessible to all. We couldn't have done this without you! We thank our publisher, Grand Central Publishing, for believing in us and for taking this idea from its raw form, step-by-step through the journey of book creation. In this regard, we especially thank Sarah Pelz and Sheila Curry Oakes for their insights and help in editing the book.

We are grateful to the Weizmann Institute of Science for providing us with the complete academic freedom to carry out research that is driven solely by our curiosity to explore the unknown in a way that we deem as most interesting. It is this boundary-free and limitless environment that allows a computer scientist and an immunologist the freedom to decide to study nutrition. The state-of-the-art infrastructure and support of our institute allows us to probe into the very secrets of life.

We are deeply thankful to the many students, postdocs, research associates, technicians, and other lab members of the Segal and Elinav labs who have joined, from across the world, this journey of studying nutrition, the microbiome, and how both interact with the human body in promoting health or the risk of disease. From secretaries, to hourly students, to autoclaving personnel, to staff scientists, you are all part of our team. Your creativity, drive, intelligence, diligence, motivation, and endless effort are driving us forward in our quest to cure human disease. We are lucky to be working with such a talented team as yourselves. The stories in this book are your stories as well.

I (Eran Segal) wish to thank Eran Elinav for being such a close collaborator and friend, and for just being there day and night, to consult and advise on both small and large issues alike. The different and complementary skills and knowledge that you bring always enrich me with a different and fresh perspective, making the end result much better and the way to get there enjoyable.

I (Eran Elinav) would like to thank my partner in crime, Eran Segal, for being a long-standing scientific partner, colleague, and, of no less importance, friend. You come from a different background and speak a different scientific language, but you make our interaction a joyful and fulfilling intellectual and personal experience.

We would both like to thank our mutual friend Professor Eran Hornstein (a third Eran!) for recognizing our common scientific interests and introducing us to each other on a cold New Haven afternoon in 2012, which was the beginning of what continues to be a long and fruitful partnership.

And last, but not least, we are deeply thankful to our beloved families. Our parents, Rachel and Yoffi Segal, and Rivka and Yankale Elinav; our wives, Keren Segal and Hila Elinav; and our children, Shira, Yoav, and Tamar Segal, and Shira, Omri, and Inbal Elinav. For too many years, we have seen far too little of you, and even less so with the making of this book. But your love, partnership, and continuous support are what make our clock (and microbiome) tick. Keren, your passion for nutrition over the past two decades, which I once ignored, has finally caught up with me and become a major part of my world. I thank you both for that and for the endless discussions and advice that you gave me on the subject. Hila, your wisdom, common sense, healthy skepticism, and (as an infectious disease specialist) your endless knowledge of microbes are always instrumental to me. We will never stop arguing about the role of microbes and human excretions (yes, at dinner; yes, in front of the children) and having a laugh while at it. Keren and Hila, we could never have done any of this without the two of you.

THE PERSONALIZED DIET

Welcome to the Future of Dieting

Imagine that there was no single food that was bad for everyone or good for everyone—not chocolate, not kale, not cookies, not a big salad, not a banana, not coffee. Imagine something you love to eat—something you think is a terrible dietary choice (but that constantly tempts you, like a juicy, fat steak or a bowl of mint-chip ice cream)—is actually okay to eat and won't have a negative impact on your health. What if a food you hate—something you force down because you think it is good for you and will help you lose weight or avoid health problems, something like rice cakes or steamed fish—is exactly the wrong thing for you? What if we told you that carb-loading with pasta before endurance sports might be bad for you and slow you down, that diet soda might be directly contributing to your weight gain, or that sushi might be making your blood sugar spike in a way that could increase your risk of diabetes?

Imagine no longer having to suffer through painful diets that restrict too many foods. Imagine never having to go through another cleanse, another "induction phase," another fast, another starvation diet. Imagine eating carbs again, eating fat again, or eating meat again, if that is what you've been longing for. And imagine not having to pay attention to the never-ending stream of confusing and contradictory dietary information telling you the foods to eat, or not eat, in order to lose weight or fight chronic disease. Imagine that science has finally begun to scratch the surface of the complex question about the optimal diet and that you no longer have to wonder what is right for you to eat, because you finally understand that there is no single correct diet philosophy that will work for all people. What if each person requires a different diet tailored to his or her own body composition? And that science is only beginning to discover a methodology so an individual can determine exactly what his or her diet should be? What if you finally understood how and why optimal nutrition must (and can) be personalized?

What if you could use that information for the benefit of your own health and weight-loss efforts, right now?

We are Dr. Eran Segal and Dr. Eran Elinav, researchers and colleagues at the Weizmann Institute of Science, an internationally renowned, multidisciplinary research institution dedicated to advancing science for humanity's benefit. We have been collaborating on an ambitious and far-ranging research effort called the Personalized Nutrition Project that we believe has the potential to shift the very foundations of nutrition science.

In *The Personalized Diet*, we will explain how we arrived at our conclusions; give you the genuine, hard science behind the surprising claims we are now able to make; and show you how you can get a jump on those changes now, in your own life and for the sake of your own health, by applying our personalized nutrition approach to the way you eat and the lifestyle choices you make. The insights we gained in our studies, based on new, large-scale data that we collected, may be life-transforming, as it may have you looking at your dietary choices in a completely new way. It's very likely that many of the foods you love, that you think you shouldn't eat, aren't harmful for you at all. It's possible that many of the foods you thought were healthy aren't good for you—not the general "you," but *you personally*. How can you know for sure? This is the future of dieting. What we discovered in our groundbreaking and internationally publicized research has the potential to change your health, your weight, your energy level, and your sleep quality—indeed, your life.

Most people want to lose weight, get healthier, feel better, and generally get control of their appetites and lower their risk for chronic disease. That's why scientists and research institutions have spent countless hours and billions of dollars researching and publishing studies to answer one simple question: *What is the best diet for humans?*

Maybe you think you know. Maybe you are already in the low-carb camp, the vegan camp, or the Mediterranean diet camp, or you have worked with a dietitian and that person has told you what to eat. In any case, perhaps you are sure science knows. After all, the question sounds straightforward and direct enough. With all the scientific advancements that have been made over the centuries, surely we know the answer to this seemingly small question by now.

The reality is that although there are many convincing books, articles, and websites written by people claiming to know the truth, many of them citing tens and sometimes hundreds of scientific studies to prove their theories, there isn't one definitive answer. Some of those who support one diet over another are doctors, or dietitians, or nutritionists, or exercise trainers, and some of them are people who have successfully lost a lot of weight and want to share how they did it. Each claims to know what *really* works, the *absolute* truth. It's no wonder that so many people flock to this kind of information, even constantly changing their opinions and strategies based on the latest thing they've read. When one diet or philosophy doesn't work, they jump to another, and then another, and then another, thinking they are being discerning because they are listening to experts.

The problem is that these books, articles, and websites all seem to champion completely different and often directly contradictory information. Even well-constructed research on any one nutritional principle or strategy can almost always easily be refuted by different research on a different nutritional principle or strategy. There are numerous studies that support or oppose every single dietary intervention available.

So, what is the real answer to the question about the best diet? Maybe science would have uncovered an irrefutable answer by now, were it not for one increasingly unavoidable reality that science is only beginning to uncover: There is no answer to the question of the perfect diet because *it is the wrong question.*

But before we get to the right question—the truly important question, and the question that actually has an answer that may transform your life—we would like to introduce ourselves.

DR. SEGAL'S STORY

Before I ever conceived of the notion of personalized nutrition, I was a scientist and a marathon runner married to a clinical dietitian. Because of my wife's profession, I was fairly certain I already knew how to eat healthfully, and I thought I made good decisions about my meals. But a few years ago, I became interested in ways I could improve my athletic performance, and in my free time, I took to researching sports physiology. This led me to start thinking about how diet might improve my performance. I wondered if adjusting what I ate could give me more energy to sustain my long runs or make me faster. If I could find good evidence for any dietary changes that might increase my speed and endurance, I was willing to try them.

Being a scientist, I am not that interested in popular literature about diet and fitness fads, so instead I turned to books with a more scientific slant, with solid research backing up their claims. I wanted to know what real, hard science had to say about the question of diet for athletic performance—specifically, my own. I respect science, and therefore I trusted science to tell me the truth. I approached this new personal project with energy and expectation, hoping to find something interesting and useful for my life.

However, the more I researched the question of how diet might help or hinder athletic performance, the more I realized that the dietary advice that was widely available for athletes (and everyone else) was often contradictory. Some of it even sounded suspiciously inaccurate. As I investigated further, I discovered, to my surprise, that the science upon which this advice was supposedly based was sometimes not up to standard, involved very small studies with only a handful of subjects, had been misinterpreted by writers and journalists, or was outdated. What at first looked like good solid science in many cases turned out to be, when more carefully examined, not very scientific at all. Most shocking to me was the discovery that the dietary advice I had always practiced (almost religiously, because I was confident that it was based in science) had no real scientific underpinnings. How could this be? How could I have missed this? How could professional curriculums about nutrition, government guidelines for diets, and nutritional advice from exercise science be based on what seemed increasingly to me to look like nothing? I had taken for granted that mainstream dietary advice was true—that is, based in proven scientific principles. The more I read, the more I realized it was not.

Many of the contradictions, misinterpretations, and especially what I perceived to be missing science had to do with dietary carbohydrates. These are the sugars, starches, and fiber in food that the body breaks down, to varying degrees, into glucose to feed the cells. Athletes think about carbs a lot. Many of us "carb-load" the night before a big athletic event like a marathon and don't worry much about eating carbs because we have been taught that carbs equal energy. Dieters often focus on carbs as well, either emphasizing them as a replacement for fat (such as with many vegetarian or low-fat diets) or eliminating them because of the belief that they are responsible for weight gain and health issues (such as with the many iterations of low-carb diets). The more I investigated, the more I saw that there was plenty of evidence both for and against carbohydrates, as well as many different approaches to carbohydrates, including some that considered them all the same and others that considered some "good" and some "bad." What was a scientist to make of all this seemingly well-researched and scientifically supported but conflicting information?

But I was still primarily interested, for personal reasons, in the exercise aspect of carbohydrates, so I decided to focus on that. For example, I read a study (this was long ago and I can't recall the source) in which people ate dates, which contain fast-digesting (or "simple") carbs, 30 to 60 minutes before running or doing intense exercise. The effect of eating these dates at first seemed inconclusive—some people eating the dates were energized and had better workouts, but others felt exhausted to the point that, a few minutes into their runs, they had no energy and had to stop. I remember stopping to think about this. Why would people respond so differently to the same food when doing the same activity at approximately the same intensity? I wondered whether this might be related to differences in how people's blood sugar levels responded to dates, because blood sugar crashes are associated with low energy. If eating dates gave one person a moderate rise in blood sugar, then that could indeed provide energy during strenuous activity. But if another person had a huge spike in blood sugar and then an imminent blood sugar drop, this could result in exhaustion. I thought about this in my own life. Sometimes I felt energized from carbohydrates, and other times I felt the opposite. Maybe you have noticed something similar in your own experience—do certain carbohydrate-rich foods give you energy while others seem to sap your strength? The more I thought about it, the more I realized that some of the foods that seemed to give me the most energy *were not always carbohydrate-heavy.* Sometimes they were foods higher in protein and/or fat. Interesting.

I decided it was time for an experiment, with myself as test subject. The first thing I tried was changing what I ate prior to my long runs (approximately twenty miles). I wanted to see what would happen if, instead of carb-loading, I ate protein and fat. The reason I tried this particular experiment was because I had heard more and more "low-carb athletes" claiming they could burn fat instead of carbs for energy and that it was even more efficient. It sounded strange, but I was curious enough to try it. I wanted to know how it might affect my physical hunger and my motivation, as well as my performance. I was a little hesitant to do this because I had always carb-loaded before exercise, eating three or four large bowls of pasta the night before a run and having a few dates or energy bars the next morning about 30 to 60 minutes before a run. I almost always felt extremely hungry about 15 to 30 minutes after my run, but I figured that was just because I had burned up all those useful carbs, and I was ready for more. After a run, I would always eat even more carb-rich foods, thinking I was responding to my body's needs. I had always believed that this was necessary to give me enough energy to run that distance, but what if I (and all those other athletes and coaches and fitness professionals I knew) was wrong?

So, one evening, instead of carb-loading, I ate a big salad with lots of fat sources like tahini, avocado, and nuts. In the morning, I set out for my twenty-mile run without eating anything (against the advice of many professional running coaches).

I was surprised at what a positive effect this diet had on both my energy level and my performance! During my run, I had just as much energy, if not more, than I had with the carb-loading.

Moreover, my ravenous postrun hunger completely disappeared. After my run, I couldn't believe that I wasn't hungry. I surmised that my body must have switched to burning fat rather than carbohydrates, and this must have been responsible for these significant changes in my energy level and hunger.

I then considered what I knew about how the human body works. When we eat carbs, we store some of that energy in our livers in the form of glycogen, for use during strenuous activity. However, we can store only 2,500 to 3,000 kilocalories' (what we typically call calories) worth of glycogen. Over the course of a twenty-mile run, it is easy to burn 2,500 calories or more, so if your source of fuel is glycogen, you can see how those stores could be depleted quickly. This could certainly trigger fatigue and postrun hunger.

Even lean people have about 60,000 Kcals (calories) of fat available for energy. This is a much bigger storehouse of energy, so it makes sense that burning fat rather than carbs is more efficient for long-term exertion. If we deplete 2,500 Kcals of fat, we consume only a small percentage of the available fat energy stores, and the need for replenishment will feel (and be) less urgent.

It all made sense to me. Switching my body from burning glycogen to burning fat on a run might finally be the answer I had been seeking. As an endurance athlete, I felt like I had hit on a eureka moment. I continued eating low carb in my daily life and noticed that I had more energy, even when I wasn't exercising. This was an unexpected benefit. I also lost some of the excess weight I was carrying, and best of all, my athletic performance steadily improved until I met my goal of running a marathon in under 3 hours: In 2013, I finished the Paris Marathon in 2:58!

Then, in 2017, I broke that 3-hour mark again running a marathon in Vienna.

As I continued with my life and athletic pursuits, I couldn't help noticing that there were some successful athletes I encountered—as well as friends and colleagues—who were not eating the way I was eating. Despite my low-carb evangelizing, some of them swore by their carb-rich diets and seemed to do just fine...even fantastically, including some vegans performing at a very high athletic level after carb-loading. Maybe my eureka moment wasn't universal. Maybe it was personal. Maybe not everyone would react to this kind of dietary adjustment the way I did. Perhaps I had found the optimal *Eran Segal Diet*, but maybe I still had not discovered the optimal *universal diet*. Based on my observations so far, I couldn't be sure.

I began to think more seriously about dietary carbohydrates. Were they, as I had previously believed, the primary and most desirable source of energy for the athlete—the across-the-board best source of fuel for the body and brain—or was a diet based on carbohydrates (even the complex type I had always thought were so valuable, such as oatmeal, pasta, and whole-grain breads) inhibiting my athletic performance, energy level, muscle growth, and brain function?

I was still in the mind-set that a diet based on complex carbohydrates as a primary energy source was good for the human body, neutral, or bad. But I kept coming back to all that contradictory research. Carbohydrates could not possibly be both good and bad.

Or could they?

That's when I thought: *Why do some people seem to thrive on diets that are high in carbohydrates, while others quickly gain excess weight or suffer from low energy? Why were some of those people who ate the dates energized and some were exhausted?* I knew people who, for example, were vegetarian and ate only fruit, vegetables, and plant foods such as legumes and whole-grain rice. They lived primarily on foods rich in carbohydrates, with relatively low levels of protein and fat. Some of them seemed to thrive, some claimed to have reversed their heart disease, and some had significant muscle and strength. Others didn't seem very healthy and were always tired and pale.

On the other hand, I also knew some "low-carb" people who didn't eat any grain-based foods or legumes and consumed hardly any fruit. They lived on green vegetables, meat, nuts, and seeds, and added fat, such as olive oil, coconut oil, and even lard. Many of them were exceptionally vigorous athletes with excellent endurance, and many were quite lean. Others gained excess body fat and suffered from dangerously high cholesterol.

How could this be? Either some of these people were lying about what they were eating—the cheating vegan secretly eating meat on the sly, or the cheating Paleo aficionado sneaking cookies and toast under dark of night—*or* some of these people were simply not responding positively, personally, to the dietary philosophy they had adopted. I didn't think the people I knew were lying about what they ate. Many of them were smart people with dietary knowledge, and they were likely to be choosing good, high-quality, high-nutrient sources of carbs, protein, and/or fat.

What else could be going on?

Perhaps, as I was beginning to suspect, it wasn't just about the food. Perhaps, it was also about the person eating the food. This led me to a completely new line of thinking, as I wondered:

What are the effects of different foods on different people?

Now *this* was an interesting and far more complex question than what I had first considered as I sought out the best foods for my exercise performance. As I began to apply myself to this new question, I considered how many factors could influence how any one person reacted to food. For example:

- As a scientist, my research focused on studying the human genome—the genetic map of the human—so I already knew that genetic differences can affect the way some people respond to food. For instance, some people are missing the DNA pieces that produce particular enzymes to digest certain foods, like milk. Maybe there were many more genetically based conditions relating to food digestion that we didn't yet understand. Is that what I was observing in the people who did or did not thrive on various diets?

- I had also been reading about the newly emerging field of science that studies the microbiome, the collection of thousands of different bacteria we all have inside our gastrointestinal system. I knew that new sequencing technologies have opened avenues of exploration into the influence of these microbes on digestion and metabolism (the way the body extracts energy from food). I wondered if different collections of gut microbes could also influence how someone might react to various types of diets, or even individual foods. That seemed a fascinating and promising area of further study as well.

- What about lifestyle? Could the level of physical activity influence the body's reaction to food? What about sleep patterns, stress levels, mental engagement? Could preexisting disease processes, age, weight and height, or the diet someone ate as a child have an impact?

If the individual, rather than the food, was the wild card, then perhaps the question of how any one person will react to any one food was too complex to answer. So how was I ever going to figure out what to eat to be a better marathoner? The more I kept coming back to my original, personal reasons for investigating these questions, the more I could feel the scientist in me getting intrigued and engaged.

But the more I read, the more I realized that there was not enough data on the subject. I knew that a data-driven approach, without prejudice or bias, was the only way to answer my questions. If I really wanted to find out more, and nobody had the answer yet, I might just have to do it myself. I would need to find something that would measure an individual response to food that would include and encompass personal genetics, individual microbiomes, and clinical parameters like blood tests, weight, and age, and lifestyle factors like physical activity, sleep, and stress. It was a lot to consider. Would such an experiment even be possible?

Because I have a background in computer science, it made sense to approach this problem by using machine learning and algorithms—basically, in these fields, we take large amounts of data and try to get computers to identify patterns and rules in the data. The interesting thing about this is that when given large amounts of data, these algorithms can identify patterns that are impossible for people to find because we can't take in and process that much information. A computer's ability to see patterns and derive rules far better than what we can see is why computers are now better than people at games like chess and the Chinese game Go.

I'd never seen this data-driven approach applied to nutrition research, but I thought, *Why not? Nutrition is a complex issue with many variables. What better way to sort it all out than with big data and a computer algorithm?* I thought this might be just the way to plug the right data into the right places to learn for sure what foods would and would not increase athletic performance, as well as improve health and support weight control, for any given person. I had no idea what information such an approach might yield, but I was already eager to find out when I met Dr. Eran Elinav.

DR. ELINAV'S STORY

I came into the world of personalized nutrition from a completely different angle than my colleague Dr. Segal. As far back as I can remember, I have been intrigued by the complexity of machines. As a child, I once opened my grandfather's transistor radio and took it apart without asking permission. I did the same with my parents' record player, only to discover a multitude of wonderfully colorful and strangely shaped metallic components, interwoven with wires. I was amazed and delighted by the complexity created by human beings just like me. Of course, after dismantling many appliances, I was left with a handful of neglected parts following my attempts at reconstruction.

But no machine compared, in my estimation, to the mysterious human body. Even as a child, I thought of the body as the ultimate complex machine, containing seemingly endless hidden parts, concealed from my eyes yet easily perceptible—the beat of my heart; the wheezing sounds my lungs would produce when I had a cold; even the feelings, dreams, and sensations emerging from my brain and nervous system. The body was a machine I couldn't take apart, of course (at least not until I got to medical school), but it occupied much of my thought and imagination. When I found my grandparents' old encyclopedia of the human body, I was elated. I spent hours flipping through the pages, gazing at the many differently shaped and colored organs, tubes, and structures perfectly fitted together. Bodies were even more complex than I realized. I wondered if I would ever truly understand them.

It was no surprise to me or to anyone around me that biology became my passion and the focus of my studies. Following a four-year military service on a submarine (another fascinating machine), I joined the Hebrew University of Jerusalem School of Medicine and finally found a place where I could attain answers to the many years of questions about the functions and intricate secrets of the human body. I embraced my studies, voraciously consuming the thousands of anatomical details I was finally able to see directly in dissection classes, the endless cellular structures I discovered through the light microscope in my histology classes, and the multitude of strange-sounding medical terms revealed to me in my pathology classes. The human machine was gradually being revealed in front of my eyes.

Yet, I found that the more I learned, the less clear the big picture became. The more I zoomed in on the intricacies of the human body, the more the rules of its function became pixilated and blurry to me. The more answers I received, the more questions I had. I felt like I must be missing something. When you take apart a record player, at some point you understand it completely. Why was the human body still so elusive?

My favorite courses were in microbiology. My professors of microbiology and infectious disease revealed a world full of hidden enemies. You can't see a virus or bacteria, but they can conquer a human, sometimes in a matter of days. A living world of tiny, strangely shaped and named invisible creatures—ordered into families and groups, including bacteria, viruses, fungi, and archaea (microbes with no cell nucleus)—was coming into focus before my eyes. This was next-level anatomy! And it was an exciting world—hostile, deadly, and obscure. My teachers were like the cavalry riding in to fight in this invisible war against our ultimate adversaries, teaching us medical students how to wield sophisticated antibiotic weaponry against our enemies, even as these foes developed resistance and emerged more potent and deadly than ever.

Next, I entered a phase of clinical practice, putting all those hours of studying, memorizing, and practicing into practical use. During these grueling years as an intern and resident in internal medicine, and as a gastroenterology fellow, I had a revelation: Even more complex than the secrets of the human body are the principles of its inner battle against dysfunction.

During this time, I was exposed to human suffering at its utmost severity. Especially troubling was a set of diseases collectively termed the *metabolic syndrome*. This included severe obesity, adult-onset diabetes, hyperlipidemia, fatty liver, and the many complications that come from all these conditions. I dealt with diabetes-associated limb amputations and blindness, kidney failure and the associated need for daily hemodialysis, heart attacks, heart failure, stroke, and sudden death. The vast majority of patients admitted to the internal medicine department where I worked suffered from this common syndrome, and the illnesses associated with it often caused severe debilitation and sometimes death. The need to deliver lifesaving cardiopulmonary resuscitation became almost a daily routine for me. This degree of suffering would have been unimaginable to me, had I not witnessed it. What was happening to people? Yet, I was surprised and disturbed that the treatments we offered these many patients, who were clearly in agony, focused on treating their many complications rather than doing anything to impact the course of their primary disease. My colleagues and I became increasingly frustrated by our inability to do anything about the vast epidemic itself and its horrible consequences. We were mopping up the mess after the fact rather than preventing the disasters before they could happen.

It was this sense of enormous failure to help my patients that, despite my years of focused study, pushed me to change directions. If I wanted to help people avoid coming to the extremes of health dysfunction, I needed to dig further into the depths of human biology, beyond the study of medicine and medical practice. Although I was already a senior physician, I decided to enroll as a graduate student at the Weizmann Institute of Science, Israel's most elite academic institution and a world-renowned center of basic science research. I would start again.

There, in the lab of Professor Zelig Eshhar, a world-famous scientist and the inventor of a promising new cancer immunotherapy, terms like *patient care*, *fluid charts*, and *medication dose* were now replaced with new terms such as *DNA*, *epigenetics*, *cytokines*, and *chemokines*. I was intrigued and bewildered by this new world but excited by what I saw as the potential to gain a deeper understanding of many of the "incurable" diseases I had encountered as a physician. Here, instead of human patients, I worked with test tubes, microscopes, and animal models. I gradually learned to combine my clinical problem-oriented medical thinking with the deep mechanistic curiosity and drive of a basic scientist. I was feeling increasingly confident that my "toolbox" was expanding and I was reaching a new level of professional maturation.

I decided to dive even deeper into science and took a postdoctoral position at Yale University in the lab of Professor Richard Flavell, one of the world's leading immunologists and cell biologists, where I was exposed to a new revolution in science and medicine that would eventually engulf me and my professional career for years to come: the study of microbes.

It was at this point that I started to think of my possible future contribution to science and medicine. What questions and topics would I pursue as an independent future researcher? For years, my teachers, colleagues, and I had considered microbes to be the ultimate enemies of human health and the invisible cause of most disease, or waste products irrelevant to our human physiology. Now I was learning that these internal microbes did much, much more. This was a new and exciting frontier in science and medicine, and there I was, on the forefront. New technologies, once regarded as science fiction, enabled us to probe deep into the nature of the trillions of microbes that live within every human body.

I was intrigued by the work of pioneers such as Jeffrey

Gordon and Rob Knight, who developed means of connecting this microbial world within a world, now termed the *microbiome*, to almost any feature of our human existence. I began to recognize that the microbiome is a significant source of health, including the prevention or cure of disease. The microbiome, I learned, was indispensable in digesting food and extracting nutrients, was an instrumental part of the human immune system, and was influential in many other biological systems. The human body is impossibly complex, and when I saw that within the body was an entire universe of microbes, I decided that this was to become my world, my mission, and the source of my contribution to science. I would be an explorer of this newfound universe, seeking the answers to the resolution of our most common and debilitating health conditions.

Finally, it was time to establish my own research group. I was fortunate to have been offered an independent position at my former graduate institution, the Weizmann Institute of Science. It was time to go back home. I established the first fully dedicated microbiome research laboratory in the institute and in Israel, established the unique infrastructure that is critically needed for this interdisciplinary research, and recruited a group of highly driven, intelligent, and ambitious students and postdocs from across the globe, who joined me in this journey that would define me and my career for years to come. Our goal: to understand how our interactions with our internal microbes affect our health and risk of disease.

It was during my transition back to the Weizmann Institute on a rainy, farewell day trip to Manhattan that I had a life-changing phone conversation. A friend, Professor Eran

Hornstein, a molecular biologist from the Weizmann Institute, suggested I meet a future colleague, Professor Eran Segal, a mathematician and computational biologist also from the Weizmann Institute. Professor Hornstein said, "Trust me, this is a great guy who has developed interests very close to yours." Trusting my friend's intuition, I arranged a phone call with Dr. Eran Segal to discuss common interests, questions, and projects we might pursue upon my arrival in Israel.

My friend was correct—the more Dr. Segal and I chatted, the more our commonalities emerged. Although our personalities were quite different, we discovered that we were distinctly complementary in our expertise, life experiences, and problem-solving approaches. We looked at research questions from different angles, used different techniques, and had different points of view, but we were both interested in the same questions: how human nutrition, environmental exposures, genetics, and immune function impact the internal microbiome and how these mysterious, poorly understood, and vastly important communications between people and their microbes impact the course of health and disease. On that rainy New York day, a partnership was formed.

OUR RESEARCH EVOLVES

Because we both had a strong common interest in nutrition and metabolism, and because our areas of knowledge were complementary, we conceived (almost from our first meeting) the idea of a massive personalized nutrition study. We were both convinced that nutrition very likely should be personalized according to each person's unique makeup, including microbiome and genetics, but we didn't yet know how. We envisioned a personal nutrition study that would be massive and wide-ranging, encompassing and controlling for a multitude of variables to discover why different people respond differently to the same foods. We knew this would be complex to design, as all good nutrition studies must be. We spent a long time on the specifics: What questions would we ask? What health measures would we consider? We wanted to measure an outcome that was important— weight loss following a diet seemed an obvious choice. However, we realized that a study focusing on weight loss alone as a primary objective to assess the effects of personalized nutrition had some problems:

1. Weight takes weeks and months to change.
2. Weight is a single measure, which might miss other important evaluations of food response.
3. Weight is influenced by many factors other than the effects of the food prescribed in a diet, such as dietary compliance, exercise level, stress level, and more.

If you go on a diet, it is very difficult to isolate the exact reason why you did, or did not, lose weight. Was it because of the addition of certain foods, or the absence of particular foods, or because of other lifestyle changes, or a combination of all these things? Which factors were influencing weight loss and which were extraneous, perhaps added or subtracted to the diet unnecessarily? As scientists, we like to design studies that allow us to isolate the effect of individual variables on an outcome of interest. We needed something that was more directly related to the food consumed, with a more immediate but also quantitative, measurable response. We wanted a metric that would be relevant for weight loss but would also be relevant for metabolic (diet-related) disease. The metric needed to be measured easily and accurately across a large study group. All of these parameters led us to consider blood glucose levels, or more precisely, blood glucose levels following a meal. We call this a *meal glucose response*, or *postprandial glucose response*—or in nontechnical language, postmeal blood sugar response.

Comparison of weight and postmeal blood glucose levels as measures of healthy nutrition

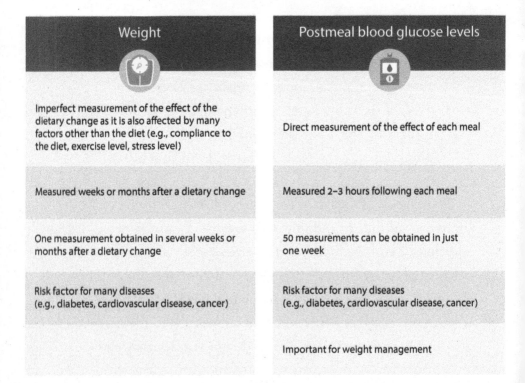

Weight	Postmeal blood glucose levels
Imperfect measurement of the effect of the dietary change as it is also affected by many factors other than the diet (e.g., compliance to the diet, exercise level, stress level)	Direct measurement of the effect of each meal
Measured weeks or months after a dietary change	Measured 2–3 hours following each meal
One measurement obtained in several weeks or months after a dietary change	50 measurements can be obtained in just one week
Risk factor for many diseases (e.g., diabetes, cardiovascular disease, cancer)	Risk factor for many diseases (e.g., diabetes, cardiovascular disease, cancer)
	Important for weight management

One reason we liked the idea of measuring blood sugar after meals was that large spikes in postmeal blood sugar promote both weight gain and hunger. After we eat, our body digests the carbohydrates in food, breaks them down into simple sugars, and releases them into the bloodstream. From that point, with the help of insulin, glucose is moved into the cells and into the liver, where it is used to synthesize glycogen, for later use as energy. But insulin also signals cells to convert excess sugar into fat and store it. This extra sugar storage is a primary reason for weight gain. Also, if too much glucose flows into the blood from food, this may cause the body to react with an overproduction of insulin; this can push glucose levels too low, even below what they were before eating. This makes us feel hungry and causes the impulse to eat more, even though we have already had enough (or more than enough) food to cover our energy needs.

We also knew that sharp glucose spikes after a meal are a risk factor for diabetes, obesity, cardiovascular disease, and other metabolic disorders. A recent study (one of many) that followed 2,000 people for more than thirty years found that higher meal glucose responses predicted higher overall mortality during the study.[1]

Finally—and this is important—recent technological advances allowed us to measure blood glucose levels continuously for an entire week. Because the average person eats approximately fifty meals per week, this technology gave us the opportunity to measure fifty meal glucose responses in one week. This would directly measure the effect of every single meal, as opposed to the more common practice of measuring someone's blood sugar once—for example, in the morning after a night fast—as the result of his or her overall diet. (Note that this technology is not widely or affordably available to everyone, but in the program in this book, we will show you how to test your own postmeal blood sugar, without having to use a continuous glucose monitor.)

Of course, we knew that there were many factors beyond blood glucose levels that influence weight and health, but we also knew it was an important one, and using it as a metric to determine food responses seemed promising and potentially informative.

Once we had hit on the metric to use, there were many small yet critical details to work out, and it took a couple of years to build the infrastructure. We were lucky to have stellar PhD students and research associates to carry out the research. We also hired people to do the logistical work, including inviting people to join the study, meeting with them, and drawing their blood. We explained how to use our app, log their meals, and collect samples from them, and we hired programmers to write the mobile apps that the test subjects would use to log foods.

We also needed to find study subjects willing to participate. We mentioned the project informally to friends, and many were intrigued by our plans and interested in the result. Some were somewhat skeptical, but we faced more interest than skepticism. The Weizmann Institute was also interested in our project, so we set up a seminar to explain our research, including our goals and motivations. We advertised the seminar by sending out mail to the Institute, hoping for at least a small audience. The room had 300 seats, but people registered so quickly that we had to close the registration—something we did not anticipate. After the seminar, approximately 100 people registered on our website to take part in the study, and after they took part, word of our study spread quickly without any advertisement. We issued invitations to register, but so many people told their friends and family that before we knew it, we had 1,000 recruits. Throughout the study, people continued to register on the website, and by the end of the study, we had 5,000 people signed up and interested in participating.

This level of response is very unusual for a clinical trial. Typically, in clinical trials, researchers work very hard to recruit participants and often must pay as an incentive. By design, we didn't want to pay because we didn't want money to be the motivation. Frankly, we were quite surprised by the response—we found that people were very eager to learn about themselves. The nature of our study required many lab tests and measurements, and participants were fascinated to know these hidden aspects of their own bodies and health. We were gratified to learn that the interest was widespread and genuine.

Later in this book, we'll explain how we set up the study, the kind of results we got, and how the app we used can help you, but for now let's skip ahead. When the study was complete, we wrote up the results in a paper that was published in *Cell* (one of the most prestigious science journals in the world), and the journal set up a virtual press conference, inviting journalists to attend. The *Cell* editors' journal suspected that interest in the research would be high, but although our previous works had received very broad international coverage, nothing could have prepared us for the response to this paper.

Within hours of the moment the paper was available to an international audience, reporting about it began to appear online and in print. Within one day, more than 100 articles were published internationally, both covering and speculating on our results. A crew from the BBC came to Israel for a week to film us. We subjected the reporter and a crew member to the same tests as those we gave to our study participants and gave them personal dietary recommendations based on their results. Our recommendations surprised the BBC reporter, but she was even more surprised when she experienced significant weight loss after following her personalized recommendations. The results were aired in the United Kingdom in prime time. As of this writing, more than 1,000 articles have appeared in major media outlets all over the world, including CNN, *Time* magazine, the *New York Times*, *Forbes*, CBS News, the *Atlantic*, and the *Independent*, as well as in the most prestigious science journals, including *Science*, *Nature*, and *Cell*.

This avalanche of publicity that caused so much excitement in major media outlets all over the world was no fluke. It was a significant and enthusiastic response to the fact that we have now demonstrated, clearly, definitively, and for the first time on a large number of people, that *individual people react differently to the same foods*. Specifically, we have shown that foods that create a healthy response in some people produce a physically and metabolically damaging effect in other people. Our study allowed us to:

1. discover exactly how people react individually to the same foods;
2. develop an algorithm that accurately predicts, based on any individual's microbiome and blood tests, the personal response of different individuals to particular foods, even before that person tried those foods; and
3. use our algorithm to provide personalized diets to people, many of whom happened to be prediabetic. The diets differed according to the individual and in most cases, when followed, normalized blood sugar levels for those who used it.

This changed everything we thought we knew about nutrition, and the implications of our discoveries are broad, providing strong evidence that general dietary advice will always be limited, because it only takes into account the food, and not the person eating it.

We believe this opens a new frontier in science and necessitates a new nutritional paradigm—a focus on *personalized* nutrition, specifically tailored not to everyone but to the individual. Now, for the first time, broad and rigorous research backs this concept. It's no longer a theory or something you have observed but haven't been able to prove, and that's significant because now this concept can finally make its way into mainstream nutritional practice and policy.

This is the new frontier of nutritional science, and we want to bring you to the front of it.

WHAT OUR RESEARCH MEANS FOR YOU

Of course, we get excited about scientific research. We're scientists, after all. And the idea that our research could end up influencing nutrition science and public policy is exciting to us. But what does that have to do with you?

Bringing our research to you in a way that you can use to your benefit is the purpose of *The Personalized Diet*. Through the lens of our own research, we will show how and why the current dietary guidelines, as well as the diet books and diet information currently available, cannot possibly be correct, and why you, as an individual, may not be able to rely on that information for your own health and diet efforts. We will explain how the science behind these recommendations cannot supply you with useful information, and why, in fact, there *cannot be* one diet or set of guidelines that is best for everyone. And we'll give you a plan so you can determine exactly what foods *you* can eat and what foods might be making weight loss or health maintenance difficult for you. The information you gain will work with any dietary philosophy you currently practice. Whether you are an omnivore or following a Paleo, low-carb, low-fat, or vegan diet, this information will personalize your plan in a way that is only relevant to you and no one else. What carbs work for you? What carbs don't? Soon you will know, just as we now know, from practicing this plan ourselves. For example, Dr. Segal discovered, after testing himself, that while he benefited from a low-carb lifestyle, there were certain carbohydrates that were fine for him, including ice cream, and he could incorporate them into his diet without any weight gain or ill effects on athletic performance. Dr. Elinav now needs to avoid bread but can eat plenty of sushi without spiking his sugar. Can you eat ice cream with impunity? Are you better off without bananas? Can you still enjoy your buttered toast and tea? Soon you will know.

We believe that *The Personalized Diet* provides a new way to think about, value, and benefit from food and provides a new set of tools for how to eat for weight loss and health. Foods and entire groups of foods are no longer "good" or "bad" for all—that croissant and cup of coffee you love might be the perfect breakfast for you, but the brown rice you have with your veggie stir-fry might be your downfall. The fatty steak might be fine, but not the tomatoes in your salad. You may very well be quite surprised at what *you* should or should not be eating. You may also finally understand why a particular diet you tried worked for someone you know but didn't work for you. Maybe you will also be relieved to learn that your so-called failures at weight loss are not your fault at all but instead the fault of information that misled you.

The Personalized Diet is science-made-accessible, presenting a new way to think about nutrition advice, and it offers practical tools you can use to determine your own path forward, so you can begin to craft an eating plan for yourself that is unique, individual, and ultimately successful at restoring your health and normal weight.

In this book, you will learn:

- **The science behind the current health crisis facing the developed world.** We'll show you what is happening, prove to you that it *is* happening, and show you how it affects you and your family.
- **What you thought you knew and why it's wrong.** Many common beliefs about nutrition and healthy eating are not science-based and are harmful to many people. We'll explain how this can be true and what the common misconceptions are.
- **What the big deal is about your microbiome.** And it is a big deal. We'll explain exactly what this internal ecosystem is really all about and why it matters so much to your health, weight, and well-being.
- **How blood sugar works.** Your blood sugar and insulin make up a complex system that responds to every food you choose to eat and to lifestyle activities like exercise and stress. This system is responsible for maintaining

stable levels of blood sugar, which is crucial for weight loss and metabolic health. We'll explain how blood sugar works, why ignoring it can lead to chronic disease, and how you can leverage it to improve your health.

- **How to personalize your meals.** Learn how to take a direct measurement of your own blood sugar to determine your personal response to your favorite foods, using a simple blood test kit available at your local drugstore or online. You'll get a tracking system, access to our free mobile app, and help analyzing your results so you can understand exactly what your results say about the foods that are right and wrong for you.

- **How to manipulate your blood sugar levels with dietary and lifestyle hacks.** Once you know how you react to certain foods, you may be able to hack your blood sugar response with the dietary and lifestyle changes we will share with you. Getting to enjoy bread again could be as simple as changing the time of day that you eat it, eating less of it, or eating it with butter.

- **How to create your own personalized diet.** Based on every-thing you discover from your blood sugar testing and what you will learn in this book, you can develop a specific, targeted nutrition strategy that is unique to your body, preferences, and lifestyle. It won't be a diet, in the sense that you won't be counting calories or feeling deprived. Instead, it will be a sensible way to eat based on your own unique responses to food. It's all about you now. What a relief, to leave all that diet dogma in the past, where it belongs, and find your own way to your ideal weight and good health. Freedom!

There is still much to learn in this exciting new field of personalized nutrition. While we don't have all the answers yet—we have just begun a great exploration into this new frontier—this is the future of weight loss and improved health. The newest nutrition research is focused on personalized diets right now, and those who are ready to embrace this concept will be on the cutting edge of an entirely new understanding about how to eat food.

And because we are scientists, you can be assured that the information in this book is based on solid science—not soft science, not poorly constructed science, but well-constructed research that has a legitimate point to make about nutrition. Unlike some diet books you may have read, we won't weigh in on anything that we don't have evidence to support. If we haven't studied it and if we do not have educated opinions, we won't try to guess the answer. We are interested in what science says about personal nutrition—and science has plenty to say to keep us all busy and moving forward into the future of dieting, where there are no longer any rules, other than those you create for yourself based on the hard data we will show you how to collect.

So back to that original question, "What is the best diet for humans?" As it turns out, that question is no longer relevant. The question worth answering has now become: "What is the best diet for *you*?" By understanding how your body responds to food, you will finally understand how to calibrate your diet for more energy, better health, lower disease risk, and weight loss that finally becomes easier than you ever thought it could be.

PART I

A Twenty-First-Century Epidemic and the Personalized Nutrition Solution

CHAPTER 1

A Bread Story

How do you decide what to eat every day? Maybe you think about it a lot, or maybe you don't, but you probably have reasons for choosing one food over another. Maybe it's about taste preference. You love carrots but you don't like broccoli. You enjoy oatmeal but you think scrambled eggs are disgusting. You can't stop eating chocolate chip cookies, but you won't touch them if they have walnuts. Or maybe you decide what to eat based on health. You try to follow the general guidelines, eating more fruits and vegetables, choosing lean meats over fatty meats and whole grains over refined grains. Or maybe you follow a very specific food plan because you want to lose weight or feel better or you think your diet plan will help you to overcome some chronic condition. Maybe you eat vegan or Paleo, low fat or low carb.

Most of us probably make our food choices based on more

than just taste preferences. We worry a lot about excess weight, health issues, energy level, or athletic performance. You might be one of the 75 percent of Americans who say they "eat healthy."[1] But is your diet as healthy as you think it is? You might be following a diet that is specifically designed to address your chronic condition or that is in line with your eating philosophy, but are you sure it is the best diet you could be eating? What would you think if we told you that healthy eating probably isn't what you think it is?

Chances are, you can't always be 100 percent sure that your food choices will make any difference at all in how much you weigh anyway. Can food influence how much energy you have, how disease-resistant you will be, or how likely you are to come down with some disease related to diet? You probably suspect it does, but how do you know if you are making the choices that will have those effects? If your dieting attempts haven't been successful in the past, you may be losing faith in the whole system.

Because we research nutrition, we hear from many people that they are disillusioned with diets they have tried. They think nothing works for them, or they just can't stick to the plans, or they have become skeptical of any health promises. If this sounds like you, we think you will be very interested in what we have recently learned, in our research, about what *you* should be, or could be, eating.

Questions about diet and its effect on health have become a driving force for some of our most surprising and unprecedented research. But before we jump ahead to our results, let's take a detour. Let's talk about bread.

BREAD: PAST AND PRESENT

Maybe you eat bread nearly every day or at least a few times per week. Maybe you eat it because you like it or because you believe it is good for you. Maybe you eat it even though you think it is bad for you. Maybe you don't eat it at all but wish you could. Is bread out of fashion? Does it deserve a comeback? Whatever you think about the "staff of life," the real question is: Is bread good or bad *for you*, and can you ever know the answer to that question for sure?

First, bread is probably the most important food on the planet, so before you dismiss it out of hand, consider that for 10,000 years, humans have milled grain and used it to bake bread. Today, billions of people worldwide consume bread in some form (e.g., loaves, flatbreads, pita, bagels, etc.), often on a daily basis.[2] Bread makes up approximately 10 percent of the calories people consume.[3] In some regions of the world, such as the Middle East, bread consumption (mostly in the form of inexpensive pita bread) may exceed 30 percent of a person's caloric intake! No matter what you think of bread (love it, hate it, or believe it to be a good or bad food), you cannot deny its pervasiveness or influence on the world.

Wheat, the grain most commonly used to make bread, has been recently vilified in some popular health books, but cultivating wheat was a key event in the Neolithic agricultural revolution,[4] and it is currently the most commonly grown grain worldwide. The United States alone produces about 750 million metric tons of wheat every year.[5]

No matter what you think or know about bread, it is true (as many claim) that bread made 10,000 years ago, or just 100 years ago, is much different from bread manufactured today. These differences are easy to discern:

1. Centuries of hybridization have made wheat an increasingly successful crop by increasing its resistance to weather and pests, but these changes in the wheat plant also impact everything we currently make from wheat, including, most prominently, bread. Additionally, modern bread has an increased gluten and starch content, a purposeful manipulation to make it more conducive to bread making.

2. Most wheat today is grown using chemical fertilizers and pesticides, unlike in the past.

3. Wheat and other grains were once milled to retain much of the bran and all of the germ, so bread flour contained many more nutrients, including fiber, B vitamins, iron, magnesium, and zinc,[6] than the highly refined white flour that is most often used in modern baking.

4. The technique used to leaven bread is completely different from what it once was. Now most bread is risen with baker's yeast, a practice that began only about 150 years ago.[7] This is a much quicker way to make bread rise than traditional methods, which used naturally fermented cultures containing wild yeast (in the air and environment, rather than from a packet), along with lactic and acetic acid bacteria.[8] This resulted in bread unique to its environment, with beneficial bacterial properties modern bread doesn't have. The closest thing we have today is naturally fermented sourdough bread, and there has been some research that showed that consuming sourdough

bread made it easier for the body to absorb minerals,[9] which is interesting because there is also research to show that modern bread decreases mineral absorption.[10]

Considering these differences, it is no surprise that there is a common assumption that ancient bread was much better for health—given its higher proportion of vitamin-rich whole grains and naturally fermented leavening agents. There is also an assumption that cheap refined bread, industrially produced from refined white flour and leavened with baker's yeast, is nutritionally inferior to artisanally produced whole-grain sourdough bread.

There are also those who believe that any bread, or indeed any product made from any grain (but especially grains containing a common, notorious protein called *gluten*, which is found in wheat, rye, and barley) is harmful to health.

But the bread haters aren't winning. Even with its supposedly compromised quality and diet trends that try to bring it down, bread remains a pervasive and popular food. Many people we know continue to eat bread as a guilty pleasure, even if they think they shouldn't, simply because they love it. Some people say that although a salad would be healthier, they prefer a sandwich or they believe eggs, fruit, or bacon to be a nutritionally superior breakfast, but they eat toast anyway. Still others champion bread but say that for bread to be healthy, it should be sprouted or made from whole grains or gluten-free grains or that it must be naturally leavened.

So, who is right? What is true? Are some breads better than others, or should we all be moving on from our global bread fixation?

As scientists, we often consider questions like these and how we might design experiments to find the answers. We have conducted research on many questions regarding nutrition, which you will learn about in this book, but one of our most interesting addressed bread. We wanted to know:

1. What happens when people eat bread in general?
2. What happens when people eat industrially produced white bread, and what happens when those same people eat the same amount of artisanal whole-grain sourdough bread?
3. Is bread a healthful food, or does its high carbohydrate content cause an unhealthy rise in blood sugar, contributing to obesity and diabetes risk?

The first step in this experiment was to review the currently available studies. As it turns out, the research on many of these questions about bread is mixed.

What We Already Know about Bread

There are some studies about bread, and they have reached some interesting conclusions. One suggested that bread consumption lowers the risk of death from any cause during the study.[11] That seems like a pretty big promise: Eat bread and you may live longer! But this was just one study, so we needed to look further.

Other studies on bread have suggested that eating bread can reduce the risk of a variety of diseases and health issues, including:

- cancer;[12]
- cardiovascular disease;[13]
- type 2 diabetes mellitus;[14] and
- metabolic syndrome.[15]

Bread has also been shown to improve:

- blood sugar control;[16]
- cholesterol levels;[17]
- blood pressure;[18]
- inflammation;[19] and
- liver function.[20]

Before you run to the kitchen to make toast or call your server to bring back the banished breadbasket, let's look at this information more critically. These studies vary in the quality and rigor of their science. There are other studies that have shown bread has very little, if any, positive or negative effect on clinical markers of health,[21,22,23,24,25] including several large-scale trials that showed no significant beneficial effect on disease markers at all.[26,27,28,29,30]

So, which is it? Is bread beneficial or not? We turned our attention to the effect bread might have on the microbiome—the community of bacteria living in the gut—because we know the state of the microbiome influences the state of health. This is a particular area of interest to us (we'll talk more about the microbiome in Chapter 5), and we wanted to know what the research revealed. There wasn't much available, but one study showed that in mice, the emulsifiers used to keep modern, industrially produced bread soft and fresh tasting altered the gut microbiome in a way that induced inflammation and obesity.[31] One mouse study is hardly reason to condemn bread, and we recognized this as an area that could benefit from further research.

We also found research specifically about sourdough bread. It said that sourdough bread not only has a positive effect on mineral absorption but also may help the body metabolize glucose better.[32] Overall, however, there wasn't much information specifically about sourdough bread either,[33] and even if there was more, it could be suspect because naturally fermented bread is highly variable, depending on the unique bacteria and fungus of the environment where it is baked. It would be very difficult to isolate which properties of any given loaf of sourdough bread were having a good or bad effect. But again, there wasn't much research. How do we know so little about such a pervasive and beloved food product? The field seemed to be open for more players, so we decided to do some experiments, teaming up with our colleague Professor Avraham Levy, a wheat expert and bread aficionado from the Weizmann Institute of Science, to help fill in the current gaps in knowledge about bread and its effect on health.

The Bread Intervention Project

We called our research the Bread Intervention Project. Our goal was to see what bread would do to people in a controlled environment, and more specifically, to see how people's bodies would react to industrially produced white bread versus artisanally produced whole-grain sourdough bread. This, we believed, would answer some of our questions and shed some light on bread's nutritional status and worthiness as the world's most popular food.

The first thing we did was choose twenty healthy people— nine men and eleven women between the ages of twenty-seven and sixty-six. None of them was currently on any sort of diet, nobody was pregnant or taking any medications currently or for the three months prior to the study, and nobody had any significant health issues, including diabetes.

Next, we randomly assigned the study participants to two different groups: One group would eat commercially produced white bread (the type often available at any local supermarket) every day for a week. The other group would eat handmade whole-grain sourdough bread every day for a week. Neither group would eat any other products made from wheat other than bread, and both groups would have only bread for breakfast and then add bread to their other meals as desired. Both groups would then take a two-week break, eating normally. Finally, the groups would switch—the group that had been eating white bread for a week would eat whole-grain sourdough bread for a week, and vice versa. During the study, we would take multiple measurements to see how the people were responding, clinically and biochemically, to the bread they were eating. We would track their blood sugar, inflammation response, nutrient absorption, and other measures of health.

For white bread, we provided people in the study with a standard popular white bread, to be sure everyone was eating the same bread. To create the sourdough bread, we hired an experienced miller to stone mill fresh hard red wheat and sift the flour to remove only the largest bran particles. We also hired an experienced artisanal baker to prepare loaves of bread using only specially milled flour, water, salt, and a mature sourdough starter, without any other additives. The dough was portioned and shaped, proofed, and baked in a stone hearth oven. Every two days, we brought this freshly baked whole-grain sourdough bread to our labs to give to the study participants. The smell was so enticing that it was difficult to keep our team members away! Knowing a losing battle when we saw one, after the second delivery, we started ordering extra loaves for our lab members.

Every person in the study ate approximately 5 ounces of sourdough or 4 ounces of white bread every morning (this translated to exactly 50 grams of available carbohydrates for each meal, just to keep it equal so it couldn't be considered a confounding factor). Everyone was also instructed to add bread to his or her other meals as much as possible. Half the mornings, everyone ate the bread plain. The other half of the mornings, they ate the bread with butter.

The amount of bread we gave the people in the study was not unreasonably large or beyond what some people might eat, but it was more bread than the people in the study were accustomed to eating—the average percentage of calories from bread consumption for the study group before the study was about 11 percent, but this intervention raised that to an average of more than 25 percent. Total calories in everyone's diets remained about the same, however.

What Bread Does to People

Once we completed the testing period, we had a lot of data to analyze. The first thing we looked at was how bread, in general, regardless of the type, affected the blood tests and microbiome of all participants in the study. The following figure is a representation of the microbiome results. Each cluster represents one person's microbiome; they are spread out around the graph because every individual has a unique microbiome configuration. The bacteria in your gut are quite different from the bacteria in anyone else's gut, and this is just a way to show that. Within each cluster, the line represents how each person's microbiome changed. As you can see, there is no pattern. Every person's unique microbi-

Shown is a lower-dimension representation of the gut microbiome composition of 20 participants

The axes are unitless and arbitrary. This is just a mathematical representation of a very complex microbiome composition that consists of hundreds of different species as a representation on two axes.

Each ellipse shows four samples (four dots) of every participant throughout the bread study, before and after eating bread #1 and before and after eating bread #2. Note that all the dots in each ellipse (i.e., all the samples of each participant) cluster, which shows that people generally retained their unique microbiome throughout the study and bread dietary intervention.

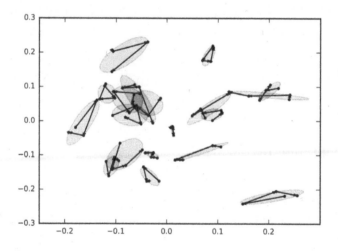

ome responded to bread in a unique way, with some more alike than others, but none were identical. Also, the changes in each person's microbiome were present and measurable, but not so significant as to change that person's overall microbiome tendency. In other words, bread affects the microbiome but does not alter it too much. By eating bread, you will change your gut bacteria, but not to the extent of transforming it to that of someone else—you will retain your personal microbiome "signature."

One pattern we saw was that, based on data we already had on long-term bread consumers, after just one week, the microbiomes of our study participants shifted in the direction of the micro-biomes of people who have been eating a lot of bread for a long time. This implies that the effect of short-term dietary changes on the microbiome is a good indicator of the effect that long-term dietary changes would have. The longer you eat that way, the more your microbiome will adapt accordingly and more permanently. But were the changes good or bad? That was less clear.

The primary information we got from this analysis was a confirmation of something we already know: We can modulate the microbiome based on what we eat. Knowing how specific foods precisely alter the microbiome is useful information. Once we know which microbiome configurations are healthier, we can then learn how to change our own microbiomes in a healthier direction using specific foods. This in turn will allow us to prescribe diets for ourselves that could improve our health just by altering our microbiomes. We believe this will continue to be an exciting area of research and new information and is an important focus of personalization.

However, at this point, as far as determining whether bread in general improved or degraded microbiome health, the jury was still out. The results were too various to make any definite conclusions—although as you will soon see, that variability would play a key role in our ultimate conclusions.

White Bread versus Sourdough Bread

The next thing we did was analyze the data that showed how people responded to industrial white bread versus handmade whole-grain sourdough bread. Like us, you probably assume that eating whole-grain sourdough bread was better for blood sugar, mineral absorption, inflammation, and other measures of health than white bread.

Our assumption was wrong. The most surprising result we observed from this research was that, on average, there was *no significant difference* between what white bread and whole-grain sourdough bread did for people—not in *any* of the clinical markers, nor in any of the microbiome features that we examined. Not in cholesterol, not in fasting glucose levels, not in blood pressure, not in weight. When we looked at our overall results, they were virtually identical for both types of bread. *Identical.* Our research results seemed to imply that all bread was pretty much the same, and it doesn't matter what kind you eat, so you might as well eat the kind you like best, or save your money and buy whatever is cheapest.

However, this finding didn't make sense to us. We thought we had to be missing something. We knew that whole-grain bread contains more nutrients, fewer chemicals and additives, and more beneficial sourdough cultures than industrially produced, preservative-filled, yeast-risen white bread. How could this not be reflected in measures of health? While we knew that our study did not follow people over a long-term period, we genuinely believed we would at least see some pattern of clinical markers edging in a good direction for the whole-grain sourdough and in a bad direction for the white bread.

We discovered we were indeed missing something! We had analyzed the averages, but averages do not express the range of responses. When we looked at the way each participant responded, we realized that the averages were hiding the really interesting story about bread. Person by person, there was a profound difference between reactions to these two types of bread—a difference that was seemingly unpredictable and, even more importantly, completely individual. The way any one person reacted to industrially produced white bread versus whole-grain sourdough was highly personal and, also interestingly, not at all in accordance with *any general nutrition theory about bread*, including theories about bread being good and theories about bread being bad. When it came to an up-close-and-personal look, none of that seemed to matter.

Upon a closer analysis, we found, as expected, some people showed more benefits from eating the whole-grain sourdough bread and more adverse effects from the white bread—but other people had *exactly the opposite response*, showing more benefits from the white bread and more adverse effects from the whole-grain sourdough bread. Some showed very dramatic effects to one versus the other, or to both, while others showed very little difference in reaction between the two. We realized that we couldn't make very many generalizations at all!

It is always confounding when the results of research are nothing like what you expect them to be, and at first, we weren't sure what to do with this data. Then again, there was one thing the seemingly random and elusive data did support—it supported our new and out-of-the-box personalized nutrition concept.

THE PERSONALIZED EFFECT

If personalized nutrition is true, that means a group of people can eat a specific carbohydrate-rich product like bread—which conventional wisdom tells us will do certain things to the body based on the food's carbohydrate content, vitamin and mineral content, and ingredient quality—and react in completely unique ways. When the food is consistent and the results are not consistent—when one person has a sharp blood sugar spike from a food that gives another person only a very mild response—that leaves only one variable: the person eating the food.

This calls into question everything we thought we knew about nutrition. If carb content, vitamin and mineral content, and ingredient quality are not necessarily related to a consistent or predictable health response, then why do those things matter? Does that mean we can all just eat whatever we want?

The short answer is no. Just because we can't predict a reaction doesn't mean you, personally, will not have a negative reaction to certain foods, so eating without any thought to health isn't going to help you and could actually hurt you. What we found, however, was that following conventional dietary wisdom, not to mention the latest fad diet, is *not* the way to discover what foods are good for you and bad for you. Maybe *you* would react positively to the whole-grain sourdough bread, and maybe you wouldn't, but until you know your own reaction, it won't do you any good to be militant about eating it or not eating it. At best, you would have a 50/50 chance that following any preconceived notions about any particular aspect of your diet would be correct. Is bread bad for you? Maybe it is, and maybe it isn't. But you aren't going to get the answer from anybody else's dietary guidelines.

So, what do we know so far? Our Bread Intervention Project confirmed a few basic principles for us that may sound completely radical up against the conventional nutritional wisdom:

1. Bread is not necessarily a bad food, and it is not necessarily a good food.
2. Without actually measuring your body's parameters, especially your postmeal blood sugar response, you cannot know for sure how you will react to bread.

But we wanted to know more. We wanted to dive into our data and really look at exactly how bread altered clinical measurements in each of our study participants. To look at personal reactions more closely, we specifically evaluated blood sugar responses. While individual responses varied over many different measures, blood sugar is generally an excellent way to determine the immediate effect of food on health, because it changes right after eating food, and it also influences and is influenced by many different clinical parameters, including age, weight, disease risk/progression, cholesterol level, blood pressure, and microbiome composition. That makes it a good general measure of individual response. We also know chronic spikes in blood sugar caused by food can damage health and increase the risk of obesity, diabetes, and heart disease, among other issues, making blood sugar a good measure of health status and disease risk. We know that a steady blood sugar, with modest and gentle rises after eating, may reduce chronic disease risk and progression. Later in this book, we will show you how to measure and analyze your own blood sugar responses to food in a similar way to what we describe here.

Overall, as we've already mentioned, there wasn't much difference between what white bread and whole-grain sourdough did to blood sugar. However, when we looked more closely, we saw that some people had quite modest blood sugar rises after eating bread, while others had larger spikes. This implies that for some people—those with only modest blood sugar rises—bread is probably a perfectly fine and harmless addition to the diet. It also implies that for those who experienced large blood sugar spikes, bread is probably not a healthy choice. This may still feel counterintuitive to you. How can bread be good for you, but not for me? And yet, this was the result we saw.

Even more interesting was the difference between breads. When comparing whole-grain sourdough bread to commercially produced white bread, we saw that again, in terms of blood sugar spikes, the differences among people were quite variable. For some, the white bread produced a higher blood sugar spike than the sourdough bread. But for others, the opposite was true. To help you visualize this, the graph below shows the blood glucose reactions to both sourdough and white bread from two different people in the study. As you can see, their reactions were essentially opposite.

Example of two participants in our study who had opposite blood glucose responses to white bread and sourdough bread

(the top participant responds more highly to sourdough, the lower to white bread)

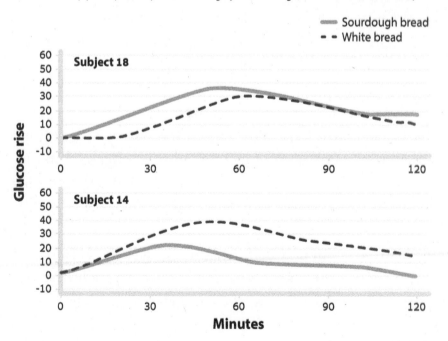

We also noticed another interesting trend: The more complex the meal, the greater the variation was in people's blood sugar response. For example, the variability across different people with plain white bread was less than the variability with white bread with butter. Sourdough bread is more complex because of its whole-grain content and fermentation products, and this resulted in even more variability than white bread with butter. We got the most variability in people's blood sugar responses with the most complex option in the study: sourdough bread with butter.

Finally, remember that figure earlier in this chapter that shows the unique microbiome configurations of our participants and their individual responses to bread? That information turned out to be quite useful because we used it to create an algorithm that could predict, using no other information but the microbiome samples, how any individual's blood sugar would respond to either type of bread. This may be something that could become quite useful in the future, as this kind of technology becomes more widely available. (We will talk much more about the microbiome and its influence in Chapter 5.)

We can form some interesting hypotheses about bread from this research, which are at the heart of *The Personalized Diet* and which will carry through to all the other research and conclusions we will cover in this book. Some of the most interesting concepts our research suggests to us are the following:

- Bread is not necessarily a healthful food for everyone. It may cause blood sugar spikes that could predispose frequent bread eaters to obesity, diabetes, and other health issues.

- Bread is not necessarily an unhealthful food for everyone. It may not cause any blood sugar problems, and it could be a good source of energy for some.
- White bread is not necessarily "bad" for some people, but it may be a poor dietary choice for some.
- Whole-grain sourdough bread is not necessarily "good" for everyone, but it may be a healthy choice for some. And, most importantly, for the purposes of this book and your overall health, wellness, weight regulation, and disease prevention, *no universal dietary rule can possibly apply to all people.*

Daniel A.

I am a graduate student at the Weizmann Institute of Science. Bread has been my favorite food ever since I can remember. As a child, the smell of baking bread was irresistible to me. When I became an adult, my quest for high-quality bread became a hobby for me and for my family. Being a "health freak," I got acquainted with the fanciest local bakeries and became a regular customer, buying a fresh loaf on my way home from a day of research. I particularly loved whole-wheat, hand-baked bread and shunned the cheap industrial white bread found in the local supermarkets. That stuff was never allowed in our house because I knew it was an inferior and unhealthy substitute for the *real* bread. This is a common belief among the people I know. I remember the uproar at my son's kindergarten when the teacher served the children white bread at lunch.

When I heard about the Bread Intervention Project, I joined up, firm in my belief in the superiority of healthy, handmade whole-grain bread. For a few weeks, I was given the delicious hand-baked sourdough bread, made from the finest and healthiest ingredients around. After a couple of weeks, I had to eat the terrible cheap white bread substitute. The sacrifices one must make for science...

Then I got my results. I was deeply surprised to see that my blood sugar responses to white bread were much lower than my responses to the healthy custom-made bread! I hoped this was a mistake, but the results were consistent for every single day I ate the "good" bread. Sure enough, it caused my blood sugar to spike, whereas the supermarket bread did not. My lucky lab mate, who also participated in the trial, had the exact opposite results than mine! Could I have been all wrong? Is there no justice?

Sadly, I have scaled back my admittedly excessive bread consumption in response to this information, but I have a new obsession now. I am completely caught up with this "personalized nutrition" concept, and I can't wait to find out what additional surprises my body (and its gut microbes) have in store for me.

What we believed prior to the study—that the health of a food was inherent to the food itself—has turned out to be only partially true. What seems to matter at least as much if not more is that unique differences in people, from health status, weight, and age to each person's individual microbiome signature, are a major determinant in how any one person's blood sugar will respond to any given food.

For you, this could mean that your approach to your own diet—the way you choose what to eat—could completely change. Foods you have been avoiding because you think they are bad for you may not actually be harmful for you at all. And foods you force yourself to eat because you think they are good for you may actually be detrimental to your health. Wouldn't that be great? As you will see, this has happened to many people in our research studies, and it has changed not just their diets but also their weight-loss efforts, health status, and lives.

Welcome to *The Personalized Diet*. We're about to introduce you to a radical new nutritional paradigm, one that has everything to do with how your food choices influence *you*. Once you understand it and know how to make it work for you, your diet may never be the same again.

CHAPTER 2

Modern (Health) Problems

Sarah and David, a couple in their midforties, are good friends of ours. They are college educated and know the standard health "rules" because they subscribe to several health magazines and watch health-related programs on television. They also discuss healthy eating tips and habits with their similarly educated friends because it is a subject that seems to interest almost everyone they know. They are both moderately overweight, but so are most of the people they know, so they don't consider weight to be a health emergency for them.

Still, they try to do what they can to lose the extra pounds. David has high blood pressure, and Sarah's doctor just told her she might be heading toward diabetes, so they do their best to avoid extra salt, fat, and sugar. They feel pretty good most of the time, except for some fatigue, and because many of their friends have the same issues, they think that their current lifestyle will probably keep them feeling good enough and hopefully living long lives.

Most mornings, they both get up early for work, despite some-times staying up too late answering work e-mails or watching their favorite shows on television. Sarah makes a pot of coffee for the two of them and puts out a bowl of artificial sweetener pack-ets for the coffee, because they are trying to cut down on their sugar consumption. They have cereal with low-fat milk because they have read that whole grains are good for breakfast and fat should be avoided. They are both satisfied that their calorie and fat gram counts are sensibly low.

Sarah works at her desk through lunch, sending out for a plain grilled chicken sandwich with no cheese or mayonnaise and some baked potato chips, while David goes out for a working lunch with colleagues and enjoys two sushi rolls with no soy sauce, to keep his sodium intake low, and a side salad with fat-free dressing. They both drink diet soda, to save even more on calories and avoid sugar.

They meet back home for dinner after their long workdays. David grills chicken, fish, or sometimes soy-based veggie burg-ers, while Sarah mixes an oil-free quinoa salad and opens a bot-tle of wine. After dinner, they watch a few hours of television. Sarah craves ice cream but tells herself that she shouldn't have any, and David longs for a bag of salty chips but doesn't want to aggravate his blood pressure.

David falls asleep in front of the television, but Sarah stays up late, straightening the house and answering more work e-mails. She goes to bed feeling hungry but also feeling virtuous because she didn't give in to her cravings for "bad" foods. She hopes that in the morning, she will be down a pound or two. She decides to weigh herself as soon as she wakes up and again after tomorrow's yoga class.

David wakes up in the middle of the night with the TV still

blaring. On his way to bed, he goes into the kitchen and eats a few slices of bread without butter or spread to quell his hunger, then lies awake in bed for another hour trying to sleep. At least he didn't break into those potato chips! He thinks that maybe tomorrow, if he's not too tired, he will go to the gym.

Sarah and David live a representative modern lifestyle. They have access to a wide variety of foods, including "decadent" foods with added fat and sugar, and "virtuous" foods that are fat-free, low sodium, or artificially sweetened. They have good jobs and expendable income. They have a comfortable home with all the modern conveniences, including health care, entertainment, and a large circle of friends and family. They also have access to technology, both for work and for pleasure, as well as for learning about anything that interests them. They have several televisions and computers, they each have a smartphone, and of course they have constant access to the Internet, to find out the answers to almost every question they have about life, health, and weight loss. Sarah and David have every opportunity. They are smart, educated, and lucky to live in this modern world.

So why is it that they are both overweight, with risk factors for serious chronic diseases?

WHAT WE KNOW ABOUT HEALTH

Most of us are lucky to be alive right now, in the twenty-first century, with its vast opportunities and resources. Never before in human history have we known as much, learned as much, or benefited as much from the products and results of human exploration, inquiry, and discovery. Since humans have first tried to understand the world around them, progress has marched on, and the longer we are at it, the more we learn. From the invention of the wheel to the discovery of gravity, from car travel to space travel, humans continue to observe, theorize, invent, innovate, and push the boundaries of knowledge.

Health and longevity are subjects in which we have advanced significantly. Humans like to study themselves, and this has resulted in better nutrition, safer environments, and the development of sophisticated pharmaceutical and surgical interventions to treat diseases and injuries. We understand what vitamins and minerals are and which ones we need in what amounts to prevent conditions such as scurvy, rickets, and anemia. We understand that calcium strengthens bones and teeth and that protein builds muscle and other tissues. We know that movement and resistance build strength and endurance, and we know that we should make ourselves move and stretch and lift heavy things to build muscle and strengthen bone. We have learned that things like seat belts in cars and caution around guns will keep more people alive, and most countries have instituted laws that encourage these practices.

To prevent and treat infections, which used to kill millions,[1] we now have antibiotics. We have a sanitary public water supply. Doctors can treat cancer with surgery, radiation therapy, chemotherapy, and lately with immunotherapy. To treat a heart attack, doctors can often repair the vessels of the heart so that it can go on to beat successfully for many more years. We take all these things for granted, although our grandparents or great-grandparents didn't have access to any of these "luxuries."

We have also discovered astounding things about how the human brain functions and ages. We have learned that every human body harbors billions of bacteria in the gastrointestinal tract, on the skin, and in every other nonsterile spot, and these bacteria have a significant effect on health and function. We have mapped the human genome, and the price of DNA sequencing has dropped over a millionfold in just over a decade (e.g., in 2001, it cost more than $1 billion to sequence the genome of one human. Today it costs less than $1,000). New technological innovations have enabled biology researchers to advance from studying single genes to studying the genetic code within entire biological systems. Many more innovative and useful scientific discoveries are on the horizon. It is an exciting time to be alive, as new discoveries happen daily.

But there is a dark side to all this progress. Considering all we have achieved and everything we know, it is perhaps surprising that we are also witnessing, along with all our advancements in health, an unprecedented dramatic worldwide rise in metabolic diseases like obesity and diabetes. Just when science has mastered so many human health issues, metabolic disease is occurring at a magnitude and scale like never before in human history.

What Is a Metabolic Disease?

A metabolic disease is any disease related to a dysfunction in the process by which the body makes energy from food. This dysfunction affects the ability of cells to perform critical biochemical reactions that involve the processing, transport, or absorption of proteins (amino acids), carbohydrates (sugars and starches), and lipids (fatty acids). This dysfunction can eventually induce a variety of biochemical imbalances, such as insulin resistance, high blood pressure, high cholesterol, and high triglyceride levels. These conditions are risk factors for obesity, diabetes, and cardiovascular disease and have also been implicated in other diseases such as cancer,[2] Alzheimer's,[3] Parkinson's,[4] and fatty liver disease.[5] In short, metabolic dysfunction puts people at risk for earlier death and poorer quality of life, just at the historical moment when science is mastering so many issues related to human health.

Metabolic disease effects and health consequences

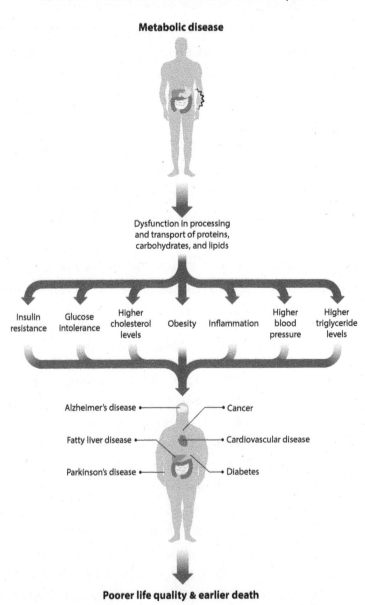

Metabolic disease is very real, and very common. If you live in the United States today, you have nearly a 70 percent chance of being overweight and nearly a 40 percent chance of being obese.[6] It's not just the United States that is getting fatter, either. Globally, obesity rates have more than doubled since 1980, and in 2014, more than 1.9 billion adults, or 39 percent of the world's population, were overweight, and 600 million of these were obese. In fact, most of the world's population now live in countries where being overweight or obese contributes to the deaths of more people than malnutrition and starvation.[7]

There is also nearly a 40 percent chance that you are prediabetic and more than a 9 percent chance that you actually have diabetes right now—a number that has nearly doubled since 2014.[8] Diabetes often goes undiagnosed for many years.[9] You are more likely to die from heart disease than for any other reason, whether you live in a developed country or anywhere else in the world.[10] The metabolic syndrome, a cluster of conditions including abdominal obesity, high cholesterol, high blood pressure, and diabetes, is practically an epidemic in the United States, with more than one-third affected since 2012,[11] and the metabolic syndrome is a known risk for cardiovascular disease.

Cardiovascular disease itself causes 17.3 million deaths per year worldwide. And if heart disease doesn't kill you, then your next likely cause of death is cancer, with more than 1,688,780 new cases expected to be diagnosed in the United States in 2017 (not including the two least invasive types of skin cancer).[12] In 2010, 33 million worldwide suffered from stroke,[13] and nonalcoholic fatty liver disease is now considered the most common liver disease in the developed world, occurring at epidemic rates.[14] Twenty percent of Americans have fatty livers, including up to 6 million children![15]

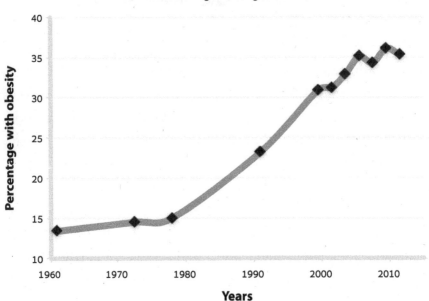

Obesity
(Percent among adults aged 20–74)

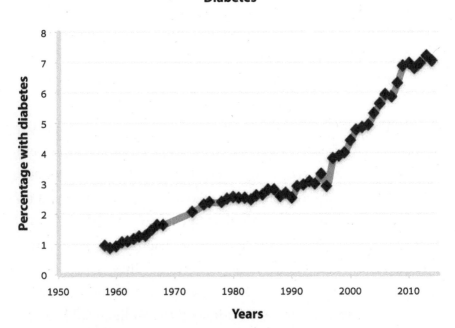

Diabetes

Neurological diseases are also a major problem in the United States. In 2016, more than 5 million Americans were suffering from Alzheimer's disease[16] and 1 million from Parkinson's disease, with about 60,000 new cases every year.[17]

This is unprecedented and very worrying. Just a century ago, the top three causes of death were pneumonia, tuberculosis, and diarrhea/enteritis. A hundred years later, they are heart disease, cancer, and stroke. In 1958, 1.6 million people in the United States had diagnosed diabetes, and today that number is 21.9 million.[18] Between 1960 and 2014, the average weight of a man in the United States increased from 166 pounds to 196 pounds, and the average weight of a woman increased from 140 pounds to 169 pounds.[19,20]

It's ironic, not to mention tragic, that in an era of vast knowledge and rapid medical advancement, we are seeing such a dramatic rise in the incidence of these metabolic diseases—diseases that so drastically compromise quality of life and that we know are preventable through simple lifestyle changes. Although gradual changes in human genetics and environmental factors that could influence gene expression could be a potential factor, it would not be influential enough to cause such dramatic changes in human health. It's true that global life expectancy has increased even since 1990, while deaths from infectious diseases continue to fall,[21] but the metabolic disease epidemic cannot be explained by extended life expectancy. There is more chronic disease incidence by age than ever before—it is not only happening in people who live into their eighties. Poignantly, the next generation is also at great risk, with more than 17 percent of American children currently suffering from obesity and related health issues, from diabetes and high cholesterol to fatty liver disease. What could

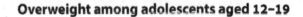

Overweight among adolescents aged 12–19

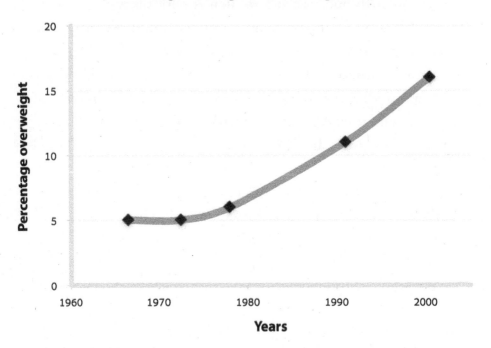

be causing the epidemic that blights our significant medical and other health accomplishments and advancements?

We think we have an answer. We believe that the very progress that has been so beneficial to humankind has also resulted in this very modern problem. Progress means change, both for the good and sometimes for the bad. We believe and will demonstrate that some of the changes we have made to our environment and way of life, due in large part to progress and our scientific, technological, and industrial advancement, have caused this rise in metabolic disease. All this ease and convenience contributes to lifestyle decisions that encourage poor health, more pollution, more artificial ingredients in food, more sedentary lifestyles, less quality sleep, and increased social isolation. Also, the rampant spread of misinformation (thanks especially to the Internet), whether based on faulty interpretations of science or faulty science itself, can result in conditions and decisions that compromise health.

But we also believe that what science has set awry, science can also fix. By examining the problem and better understanding the obstacles we face, we are confident that we can find solutions.

Guy R.

I heard about the Weizmann study on personalized nutrition through my wife and decided to register and take part in it. I was overweight but did not know about any other health issues that I had. After the study, I was told that my blood sugar responses were abnormal and were in the prediabetic range. I also found that many of the foods I normally eat, such as pita bread and rice, spike my glucose levels but that other foods I enjoy, like beer, chocolate, and hummus, did not. I received a menu based on my test results, which I followed. I was surprised by how easy it was, probably because it allowed me to eat many of the foods that I love. Within a few weeks, I lost 20 pounds and returned to my normal weight, and my blood tests showed that my glucose levels were back to a normal, non-prediabetic range. This has completely changed my eating habits and probably saved me from developing diabetes!

Twenty-First-Century Lifestyle Changes—New and Improved?

We don't romanticize the past—we are proud to be on the forefront of scientific advancement. But we have also specifically studied how certain aspects of modern life have resulted in health problems. Let's set the stage by looking at some of the lifestyle changes we have all experienced—that don't have anything to do with diet—to see what they are doing to us and what we might do about it.

How Sleep Has Changed

We don't sleep the way we used to sleep. In fact, modern sleep patterns are markedly different from those of our ancestors, who were active as long as sunlight was present, then spent a few quiet hours by firelight after sunset, followed by a long sleep until the sun rose again. This pattern of complying with the light–dark cycle existed for millions of years and dictated the development of every living system. However, for fewer than 200 years—a fraction of time on the scale of human history—we have been living with electric lights and long-distance travel, no longer dependent on natural light cycles. This rapid and dramatic change has disrupted our circadian rhythms, or the natural sleep/wake cycle that exists in all the cells and organs of our body. This disruption has resulted in some major health issues, and it all began with the electric light.

What Is Circadian Rhythm?

Circadian rhythm is the internal rhythm, or sleep-wake-eat cycle, of all living things (humans, animals, even plants and bacteria). It is linked to the 24-hour cycle of the sun, and it is based on exposure to light. Humans (and other animals) have innate mechanisms for sensing light, primarily detected by the retina,[22] which signals the brain to influence these internal "clocks."[23] This is why people tend to get tired in darkness and wakeful in the light (the pattern is the opposite for some nocturnal animals). Amazingly, our brains have these "ticking clocks" regulating our bodily behavior, and in the past two decades, science has discovered that every cell and organ in our body features a clock of its own.[24] We therefore have millions of clocks ticking in our body at all times, perfectly coordinated with one another to perform just the right activities during different times of day. Collectively, the brain clock (termed the *central clock*) and all the millions of our other clocks (termed *peripheral clocks*) determine our healthy circadian rhythmicity.

Circadian rhythms influence us in many ways, from internal biochemical changes that signal sleep/wake behaviors, to the way we've constructed our entire human society—most of us get up in the morning, go to work in the light, and when the sun goes down, we start thinking about going to bed. Circadian rhythms are individual and can be driven by genetics and behavior but are also amenable to major changes coming from our environment. For example, suddenly changing your habits (like taking a long-distance flight across time zones) induces severe disturbances to your circadian rhythm, but after a while, your body adjusts to the new environmental light–dark pattern and resumes its normal circadian rhythms. In contrast, people working night shifts constantly change their environment in a way that makes it impossible for their bodies to adjust the circadian rhythm. Even if they work during the night and sleep during the day, they will be exposed to opposing natural light cycles. Living in such a circadian-disturbed fashion for long periods of time has been shown, in our research and the research of others, to predispose people to severe health issues.

The way we work and sleep is far removed from how our ancestors lived, when the only evening light was firelight or candlelight and the morning came without blackout shades and sleep masks. We, in contrast, have electric lights to make our living environments bright as midday, even in the middle of the night. We have TV screens, computer screens, and smartphone screens to keep our eyes focused on light and our brains engaged in work or socializing, at a time when our ancestors would have been long asleep. Since the invention of the lightbulb in 1879, our reliance on the sun has become less and less necessary, culturally if not biologically. We are no longer as compelled to live according to our circadian rhythms. We have power over our environmental lighting (or does it have power over us?). Moreover, we are now able to reverse our light–dark environment within hours, by engaging in long-distance travel. While the resultant jet lag is uneasy but usually tolerable, frequent flyers are exposed to exactly the same circadian-rhythm disturbances and associated health risks as shift workers.

Sure, we get a lot more done this way, and our social lives are probably more interesting. But there is a price for the convenience that allows us to do what we want at any time of day or night. Light—any light, whether from the sun or electric lights or screens—interferes with melatonin production.[25]

How Your Brain Puts You to Sleep

Melatonin is a hormone secreted by the pineal gland in your brain that helps to regulate sleep and waking, as well as the cycles of other bodily functions. Brain function and sleep cycles use some of the same neurotransmitter systems, so when sleep is disrupted, it can affect cognitive ability and metabolic function.[26] Some people take melatonin supplements to help them sleep, but whether or not this can come close to mimicking what happens with natural exposure to sunlight and darkness is questionable.[27] Some people say it works for them, but there is not, as yet, any hard, scientific proof of this.

Like a snowball growing bigger as it rolls down a hill, disrupting melatonin production disrupts circadian rhythm, which disrupts a cascade of hormone-related processes, which in turn could eventually lead to disease and dysfunction. For example, circadian disruption in people engaged in prolonged shift work (such as physicians, nurses, and soldiers) has been linked to increased breast cancer incidence, likely due to how circadian rhythm disruption affects estrogen production and estrogen receptor function.[28,29,30] Psychiatric and neurodegenerative diseases, like depression and dementia, are also closely linked with disrupted sleep cycles,[31] and circadian rhythm disruption has also been tied to a higher incidence of major depressive disorder[32] and some other types of depression.[33] Immunity, cardiovascular disease, and many other health issues[34] are also more likely in cases of circadian rhythm disruption. Most prevalently, people having a lifestyle involving chronically disturbed sleep/wake cycles feature a very significant risk of developing obesity, adult-onset diabetes, and their complications.[35,36]

The question of how circadian-rhythm disruption influences health interested us, and we conducted our own research on the subject, specifically looking at the microbiome (and bacteria within the human gut, which we will talk about in more detail in Chapter 5) and how it responds to circadian-rhythm disruption.[37] We studied mice undergoing conditions that mimic severe jet lag, by changing their lighting conditions and feeding patterns, to disrupt their circadian rhythm. We also studied people undergoing actual jet lag. The results were interesting. We will talk about these studies in more detail, but one of the most fascinating findings was that the microbiome itself—the collection of bacteria in the gut—follows a circadian cycle all its own, which is synchronized to the clock of the person. In other words, you are influenced by your own circadian rhythm, as well as the synchronized circadian rhythm of the bacteria living in your intestines.[38]

We know there is also a genetic component to this issue. We have already discovered in our own research that there are genes in our cells that act as clocks. We found that if you delete these genes in a mouse, then the rhythmicity of the microbiome is lost. It seems these internal clocks are both influenced by multiple parameters and influence multiple health issues.

Therefore, disrupting your circadian rhythm disrupts the circadian rhythm of the bacteria in your microbiome, and that seems to be a primary cause of the glucose intolerance and obesity we see associated with circadian-rhythm disruption. Because people with jet lag experience similar disruptions to those of shift workers who work during the night and sleep during the day (essentially giving themselves jet lag without going anywhere), we believe this may explain why so many shift workers suffer from these metabolic diseases.[39] Eating at night can also cause this disruption (something shift workers must do). In our research, we showed that when we shift the eating time of mice to daytime (mice normally eat at night), then their microbiome rhythmicity is also disrupted.

In other words, both the genetics and the lifestyle (jet lag, shift work, night eating) of the host (the mouse or the person) can disrupt circadian rhythm and influence microbiome

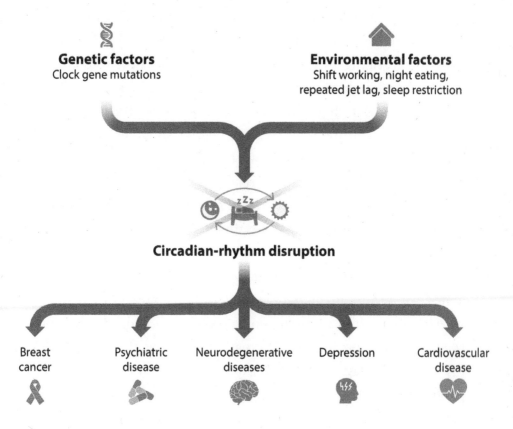

Circadian rhythm and possible effects on health that its disruption could cause

rhythmicity—and disrupting your microbes' normal daylight behavior can have severe consequences on your health.

The Blue-Light Disruption

Light disrupts circadian rhythm, but the color of light affects how severe that disruption will be. Prior to the proliferation of electricity, light mostly came from the sun or fire, which contains more red light waves. Now, most of the light we are exposed to comes from lightbulbs and, increasingly, screens of computers and other electronic devices, which contain more blue light waves. Consider that 90 percent of Americans report using some form of technology in the hours before bedtime.[40] Because blue light suppresses melatonin production more than other forms of light,[41] electric lights and screens are more disruptive to circadian rhythm. Light that is composed more of red waves, such as candlelight and firelight, does not have this same effect and does not induce wakefulness to the same degree, so its disruptions to circadian rhythm are milder. Two hundred years ago, when our ancestors stayed up past sunset reading or socializing by candlelight or a roaring fire, this likely did not interfere with circadian rhythms the way lying in bed texting or Googling or reading an e-reader or watching television can do now.

Finally, consider how often we now travel between time zones, something many people, including us, now do regularly. In 2015, more than 1 billion people traveled abroad,[42] compared to just 25 million in 1950,[43] greatly increasing the worldwide influence of jet lag on circadian rhythm. Research shows chronic jet lag could influence multiple health mechanisms, from memory and cognitive function[44] to tumor progression.[45]

What are you supposed to do if you must work the night shift or travel cross-country or to other continents regularly? What do you do if you think you are addicted to television time or your computer or smartphone? Some of these things may be under your control, and some may not, but understanding what is happening when you get too far away from waking and sleeping in synch with the sun can help you understand your disease risks. Whether you decide to do anything about it is, of course, up to you. There isn't any convincing evidence, in our opinion, that any therapies can make those disrupting behaviors less disruptive—you may have heard of "remedies" like melatonin supplements and blue-light-blocking screens and glasses, but the proof just isn't there. Of course, you can try them if you like, but in our estimation, your best strategy is to get back in synch with your natural rhythms as much as is possible and realistic in your life and to keep track of how and when you sleep to help you be more cognizant of how you are choosing to keep your schedule.

Exercise and Sedentary Behavior

Can we get away with eating more if we exercise more? Maybe, but the problem is, most of us don't move enough throughout our day to make a difference. Prior to the Industrial Revolution, most jobs involved relatively intense physical labor. Then along came machines, and then more advanced machines, which replaced many labor jobs. And then came computers.

Even an hour a day at the gym before or after your desk job can't compare to the level of physical exertion of a manual labor job, let alone the exertion it would take to hunt for food, build a shelter, or walk for miles to get water or interact with other human beings. Obviously, there are still many people performing manual labor jobs, and they may be somewhat less prone to metabolic disease, all other things being equal.

Here too, progress in general has been beneficial. We easily produce goods and services that were never available before, and we can travel pretty much anywhere without much effort in cars and airplanes, so far fewer people today have to exert themselves physically. Working is generally much less hazardous than it once was. In the past, many people suffered physical harm from harsh workplace environments and accidents. Many worked as farmers, loggers, miners, and fishermen, as well as in manufacturing, with few if any safeguards. Only relatively recently have we had protective labor laws and child labor laws and a prioritization of safety.[46] That's all good news. Even now, research shows that while physical activity is good, hard manual labor is linked to a higher risk of heart disease.[47] Working too hard is dangerous.

Nowadays, most Americans work at desks. In 1970, 20 percent of Americans worked at desk jobs or jobs that required minimal activity, while 30 percent of Americans held jobs that were physically taxing. Just thirty years later, 40 percent of U.S. adults had jobs that required very little activity, while only 20 percent had physically taxing jobs.

But recent research has highlighted the dangers of sitting too much, calling sitting "the new smoking"[48] because the more people sit, the more likely they are, the research says, to develop diabetes, heart disease, and obesity. They may even live shorter lives.

Also, we spend time looking at those ubiquitous screens. In just the last twenty years, both the availability of screens and the time we spend gazing at them have increased dramatically. In 1989, just 15 percent of households had computers with Internet access. In 2009, that number rose to 69 percent. For most of us, a hard day's work means sitting in front of a computer, at a desk, for 8 or more hours, with a lunch break in the middle, and most of us know we should be moving more, not less. At the end of the day, most of us sit more—in front of televisions or back at our computers for surfing the Net or social networking or on couches with our smartphones.

While this constant screen time likely has a psychological

effect on modern culture, the physical effect is obvious. Sedentary living leads to health risks.[49] Research has shown a direct correlation between hours sitting each day and larger waist circumference, higher fasting triglyceride levels, and insulin resistance.[50]

"But I Have the Fat Gene!"

You are born with your genes, mutations and all, and those don't change. However, that doesn't mean genes are destiny or will necessarily correspond with any particular health outcome.

Genes are a risk factor for certain diseases and/or conditions, such as obesity. They indicate a tendency, but they do not predict a destiny. Just a few dozen years ago, some conditions such as obesity and diabetes were much less prevalent globally, and our genes have not changed in this very short time frame. Instead, health and weight are ultimately the result of the combined effect of multiple factors: your external environment, your internal environment (including your microbiome), and epigenetics, or whether your genes are activated by your environment and to what extent.

Each of these affects the other, back and forth, in a dance of influence that ultimately determines your weight, health, and whether you will or will not develop any disease:

- Genetics influences disease risk. Your DNA determines which mutations and which variants of each gene you are born with, and that can influence gene function. For example, you may have a mutation in the gene responsible for producing the enzyme that breaks down lactose, and that could cause you to become lactose intolerant. But if you consume little or no lactose, this tendency will never show up.

- Genetics influences the microbiome—although not as much as you might think. Recent studies (including our own) show that to a certain extent, genetics determines the composition of the microbiome. For instance, identical twins tend to have somewhat more similar microbiomes than fraternal twins,[51] which have more similar microbiomes than siblings, which have more similar microbiomes than unrelated individuals do. However, we were surprised to find how small that influence really is.
- Genetics influences epigenetics. It is well established that our DNA encodes the programs that determine when, where, and to what extent genes will be activated in the body.
- Environment influences the microbiome. Research shows that people with different dietary habits (diet is a good example of environment) have distinct microbiomes. We know bacteria are fed by what we eat, and thus nutritional input necessarily drives microbiome configurations to a large extent.
- Environment influences epigenetics. We know that our environments and behavior—for example, temperature, seasons, sleep, and physical activity—all influence gene activity.
- The microbiome and epigenetics influence each other. The bacteria in the microbiome produce molecules and metabolites (smaller molecules) that affect gene activity. In turn, gene activity produces metabolites that affect bacterial activity.
- The microbiome and epigenetics influence metabolic disease risk. This back-and-forth interplay of metabolites produced by the microbiome and the genes also influences metabolic processes in the body, including those that can increase metabolic disease risk, such as fat storage, fat utilization, and fat breakdown.

Interplay and effects of different factors on metabolic disease

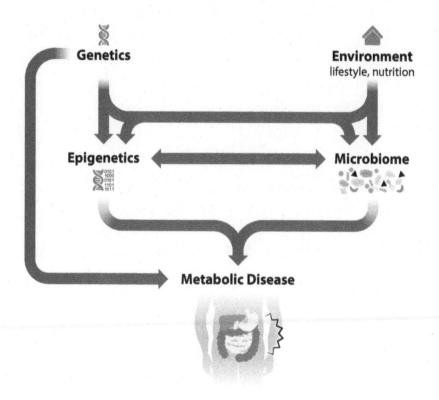

It's Cheap, It's Plentiful... but Is It Food?

So far, we haven't been talking about food, and we have a lot to say in the next chapter about nutrition misconceptions, but let's also consider how much our food system has changed, in the name of progress and the goal of feeding a large population efficiently and cheaply. We are talking about industrial food production, and while this high-tech (and highly profitable) system has resulted in lots of cheap food for everyone, it has also resulted in a well-documented decrease in the quality and purity of food.

One thing we can say for this system: It is efficient. We no longer have to eat only what is currently in season, nor do we have to rely on what can be grown only in our immediate area. We can easily buy food from other countries and food that is not locally in season, any time, at our local supermarkets—oranges from Florida, avocados from Mexico, bananas from South America, cherry tomatoes from Israel, or mandarin oranges from Spain.

We Eat More

In developed countries, the majority of people take in more calories than they need to fuel their largely sedentary lifestyles.[52] Worldwide, in the years between 1964 and 1966, the average person consumed 2,358 Kcals per day. In 2015, that number jumped to 2,940. In industrialized countries, that number has increased from 2,947 in 1964 to 1966 to 3,440 Kcals in 2015. Although the notion of calories being directly equivalent to weight gain or loss is problematic, we are experiencing consumption of almost 180,000 more calories every year.

In fact, most of the foods we eat today are probably not produced locally. Local food is so rare that it has become a fad, with some supermarkets and health food stores featuring it as a rarity for the privileged few to afford. Even those who try to eat locally now aren't usually able to do so 100 percent of the time, unless they want to limit their choices drastically. While there is not much research on the impact of this nonseasonal and nonlocal change in food patterns, it is obviously a significant change that could already be having an impact on what we eat and what our bodies (and microbiomes) do with that food.

Another crucial aspect of the industrial food system is a change in the very nature of the food itself. Due to hybridization and manipulation of food to increase yield, improve taste and appearance, and help food to withstand cross-country or inter-continental travel, most popular foods have been transformed significantly in the last hundred years in a variety of ways. For example, to produce more meat more efficiently, animals bred for meat often live in close quarters with hundreds or sometimes thousands of other animals. Those close quarters make the animals more prone to infections, so they are frequently given antibiotics to prevent disease and death. In the United States, cows are often given hormones to increase milk production or muscle size (although due to public pressure over antibiotics, farmers are increasingly opting not to do this). Animals are also bred for more milk and meat production so that, after multiple generations of selective breeding, the animals often look much different than they looked in previous generations—fatter, with much larger muscles, larger udders, and taller hind ends to accommodate milking machines.

Animals aren't the only food sources to be manipulated. Popular plant foods that are easy to grow in large quantities, like corn, soy, and wheat, are ubiquitous in our food supply and have been purposely bred over time to contain more starch and less chaff and to have a sweeter taste. These foods have also been broken up into ingredients like high fructose corn syrup, wheat starch, and soy protein isolate and then used to add sweetness, body, carbohydrates, and protein to processed foods. Plants are also routinely treated with pesticides, to minimize insect damage and maximize yields. These changes result in more food that lasts longer on the shelf and tastes good, but this level of processing is so recent that we don't yet fully understand how it will influence human health.

If we are getting enough protein, carbohydrates, and fat, and we don't eat too much, does it really matter what alterations are made in the growth and manufacture of our food? The answer is unknown. Unfortunately, there has not been much research aimed at measuring the isolated effects of each one of these changes and what impact they have on health. But because they are indeed very large changes, we think it is safe to say that the potential impact—whether negative or positive or both—is significant.

CHAPTER 3

The Misinformation Highway

There is another change in the modern world that has to do with health but that is quite different from other types of progress because it is more pervasive and less obvious. We believe it is so important to be aware of this issue that we have devoted a chapter to the topic. Before you read another scientific study or, more importantly, another article or blog based on a scientific study, we hope you will read and digest this concept: You can't always trust what you read, hear, or think you know.

In our modern world, information is king, but we think it might be more accurate to say that misinformation has captured the castle. We won't go so far as to say that the dissemination of information has ever been without issues, but in this day and age, it is very hard to discern truth, whether that applies to world events or politics or local news stories or, as is our focus, nutrition science.

Information is more available than it has ever been before,

and this has benefited general knowledge. For example, patients know more about their medical conditions than previously, because there are so many accessible resources for people to learn about health. But precisely because so many people seek health, medical, and nutritional information on the Internet, we think it is important to understand how to best evaluate and use the information you may find there.

The first thing to understand is that science is on the job. Scientists know, understand, and have studied many aspects of health, disease, and nutrition. But there remain many unanswered questions. Science is not finished. Unfortunately, unanswered questions do not make popular headlines or clickbait, so there is a tendency to create the impression that science has answers that are more finite and complete and widely applicable than they actually are.

It's easy to see how this can happen. Studies are specific to their own research subjects. Results that are relevant to a particular group of people or animals studied under a prescribed set of circumstances and over a set amount of time cannot necessarily be applied to the whole population. For example, a mouse study might shed some light on a process in humans—or it might not. If a group of mice in a study lost weight on a low-fat diet, for example, that does not mean all people will lose weight on a low-fat diet. Some might, but this kind of research does not mean we know anything definitively.

For this reason, most studies include some kind of caveat explaining the limitations or asserting that the theory will require further study. Anyone can certainly speculate a research conclusion applies more broadly than the study itself or is now a fact because research supports it, but that is different from proof.

The smaller the study and the more unlike humans the subjects are (such as mice or fruit flies), the less likely the results can be definitively applied to people in general. Knowing something conclusively is a long and complex process. Unless the study is in humans and is very large-scale (and even then), it is only hypothesis, not a fact. However, because we like simple, take-home messages and rules that tell us what to do, the media responds to new findings by making even tentative research results sound as if they are facts and apply to everyone. Here is how this can happen:

- **Research is sometimes rushed.** While in most cases, researchers do their best to publish their findings only when their studies are completed and properly analyzed (to the best of their ability), in some cases, they are pressed to publish their studies even when premature, as their funding and promotion often depend on these publications. In most but not all cases, scientific works are subject to an anonymous peer-review process.
- **Scientific publications are not all equally rigorous.** Researchers publish their work as a paper in a scientific journal explaining their process and conclusions. Scientific journals greatly differ from one another with respect to their quality and rigorous editing and publication policies, but these differences are often disregarded by the general media.
- **Press releases can simplify or overinterpret published research.** Research publications are often considered a university's display window and an effective way to attract philanthropists. Once scientific research is published, the researcher's institute or university often writes a press release about the work, and there is usually pressure by

the institute's PR team to simplify the story and give a bottom-line message. This creates a great temptation to generalize and simplify the results in a way that may not be completely accurate and may even be over-interpretive.

- **The media often hypes what sounds like a good story.** Journalists receive the press releases and generalize results even further to make good stories with good headlines. In many cases, the journalists haven't read the original study. They work only from the press release.

- **Good stories spread quickly in the media and are often changed along the way.** If the story sounds really interesting, then other journalists will further paraphrase the first round of journalists without even reading the original press release, let alone the original paper.

- **Nutrition hysteria in particular is contagious.** In the field of nutrition, which is a focus of interest for most people, this "chain reaction" is most pronounced, often leading to a serial headline production of findings that are inaccurate, to say the least. In some uncommon cases, press releases are being issued even prior to the scientific peer review process and publication, leading to unfounded mass hysteria. A classic example of this tendency was an article about a study that showed that in a test tube, acrylamide may feature carcinogenic properties. The story spread through the media like wildfire in 2002, claiming that common foods like French fries and rice that contain acrylamide could cause cancer. This was a gross overstatement, but the exciting headlines were everywhere for a short time, causing mass hysteria without real substance.

Observational versus Interventional Research

The more you understand how different types of scientific research work, the more you can critically analyze the truth behind the conclusions. There are two major types of research studies. Observational studies (also called *epidemiological studies*) are done across large populations—hundreds, sometimes many thousands of subjects—and often over large amounts of time, following subjects for months or years or even decades. These can show interesting trends, but they are also full of confounding factors—other things that could be influencing the results because the large population and long time period make it much harder to isolate the effect of one parameter over others.

The other type is interventional studies. These are more tightly controlled, so they are better at showing causality (that the intervention directly causes a change). However, these are usually very small studies, sometimes only ten or twenty subjects—rarely one hundred or two hundred, and even these are considered small. Also, interventional studies are usually designed to show the benefit of an intervention, so any deductions about harmful effects are not usually the focus of the study and may not be as controlled. In other words, interventional studies are better suited to showing that something works, rather than that something doesn't work, and although these are less likely to have confounding factors, it is much harder to generalize the results to a large population.

INDUSTRY INTERESTS

When money is involved, it can get even more difficult to discern what is and is not true. When billions of dollars are involved, the stakes are even higher. Unfortunately, there is a lot of money in science, especially when industry is involved in funding research. If a wealthy industry pays scientists to do a study, hoping for a positive result regarding the industry's product (whether a food product, a drug, or something else), there is a lot of pressure on scientists to arrive at the result the funding industry is looking for.

A good example of this bias is a report that recently emerged showing that in the 1960s, the sugar industry group Sugar Research Foundation (now known as the Sugar Association) paid three Harvard scientists to skew a review of research into the effects of sugar and fat on heart health, to emphasize the role of saturated fat and deemphasize the role of sugar.[1] The review, published in the *New England Journal of Medicine*,[2] was probably influential in boosting the idea, still widely believed today, that dietary fat and not sugar is the primary cause of heart disease, although there is scant evidence that dietary fat alone can be implicated in heart disease.

One of these paid-off scientists was D. Mark Hegsted, who later became the head of nutrition at the U.S. Department of Agriculture, where he helped to draft one of the first documents to lay the groundwork for the U.S. dietary guidelines[3]—a document that has never existed, in any of its incarnations, without industry influence.[4] Imagine if you had to create a document advising an entire country about what to eat, but people who make a lot of money selling every food product you may or may not recommend is on your advisory committee.

This influence on research happens all the time. In 2015, the story broke that Coca-Cola, one of the world's largest beverage producers, had teamed up with a group of scientists to spread the word that sugar had very little to do with obesity and was really only implicated significantly with tooth decay.[5] Another example: A study with the surprising bottom-line message that children who eat candy tend to weigh less than children who don't just happened to be underwritten by candy corporations.[6] Every scientist knows that when the people funding their research have a vested interest in the results of that research, there is pressure on the scientists to produce a headline-worthy conclusion that is in the best interest of the sponsor's bottom line. It's all about the money. Not public health.

Food Politics

If you are interested in the politics of food and the effects of food industry interests on science, a great source of information is Marion Nestle. You can find her blog and links to her books at www.foodpolitics.com. Marion keeps track of how many of the studies that were funded by the food industry ultimately supported that industry's cause. At the time of this writing, the most recent update put the score at 156 supporting, 12 not supporting.[7] This may not be surprising, but it certainly does not increase confidence in the science!

FAULTY SCIENCE

Finally, there are issues with the quality of some scientific research that can influence the reliability of scientific conclusions. Beyond pressures from the media and industry, scientists don't always have all the information they need or, being human, may sometimes design studies that don't consider important influences. There are many ways research can be faulty or turn out to be faulty when further research emerges. Nutrition science is difficult because the nature of nutrition makes it hard to construct a study with reliable conclusions that apply to everyone. There are several reasons why:

Scientists can't do studies for free. Somebody has to pay for them. If you want to do a large study, using perhaps tens or hundreds of thousands of people, you can't make the actual study too complex, or the cost would be prohibitive. Numbers of participants drive up cost. You might only be able to measure a few things like age, gender, or body mass index (BMI), or you might have to rely on people to self-report what they ate, which can be inaccurate, especially in a large group. However, studies with limited measures like this don't usually turn out to be very informative.

The other option, to meet budget, is to study more parameters but in fewer people. A study of this type might examine the effects of a dietary intervention, like low fat versus low carb, but on a group of perhaps only ten or certainly fewer than fifty subjects. This also makes the results potentially less useful or indicative of what would apply to a large group of people. Even in studies like these, there usually isn't money for true feeding experiments, in which the researchers provide all the food so they can directly control what people are eating. The people in the study are typically instructed on what to eat, and they eat on their own without any supervision by the researchers. They may not know exactly how to follow the diet, or they may not follow it according to the directions. If there is no objective measure of how closely people actually adhered to the diet, then the conclusions will not be reliable.

Food is complex. Imagine a study about low-fat versus low-carb diets. If you tell participants to eat a low-fat or low-carb diet, they will probably do what they think they are supposed to do, but it would be very difficult to completely control for those macronutrients. Many vegetables contain some fat and some carbs. Whole grains contain fat. Pure meat doesn't contain carbs, but meat mixed with anything else does. And what is the meaning of "low"? You could count carb or fat grams but you can't always control what people are actually going to eat, what they are going to tell you they are eating, or what they think is correct to eat, unless you keep those people in an isolated environment and completely control everything they eat. But that isn't a very good measure of real life, either, so the results may not be useful. You can never actually completely isolate those nutrients. Also, studies sometimes claim results based on certain kinds of foods, but if you look at the actual foods eaten, you can see the problem. For example, many mouse nutrition studies feed high-fat mouse chow to make mice gain weight, and report that they fed this "high-fat chow," but high-fat mouse chow is also very high in sugars. So, was it the fat making the mice gain weight or the carbohydrates from the sugar? If mouse chow is complex, imagine how potentially confusing it can be to look at the diverse human diet.

Health and weight are complex. There are many factors that affect health outcomes, including weight, over a long-term period. It is extremely difficult to isolate the effects of individual components on health or weight, and to conclude otherwise is irresponsible. For example, if someone loses weight on a low-carb diet, can we be sure it was the reduced amount of carbohydrates in the food or a combination of many factors, and can we then extrapolate that information to the general population? The dirty little secret is that usually we can't. Yet, the media knows we want to hear what will help us lose weight, so again, they generalize or make assumptions that are suggested but not definitively confirmed by the research. When these faulty conclusions, whether committed by the scientists, their institutions, or the media, affect mainstream health behaviors and governmental policy (such as the creation of the food pyramid; see page 99), then this can be dangerous for public health.

Science advances. Science is not just a numbers game. You may also regard it as an art form. Einstein said, "The formulation of a problem is often more essential than its solution, which may be merely a matter of mathematical or experimental skill. To raise new questions, new problems, to regard old problems from a new angle, requires creative imagination and marks real advances in science."[8] Everyone knows science once "proved" the world was flat and the sun revolved around the earth, until someone dared to challenge these views and, using newer, more advanced scientific techniques, proved otherwise.

Although we now know the earth is round, as scientists, we don't quite see it as a "mistake" that scientists once thought it was flat. The scientific method is straightforward: You collect data, and then you use that data to build a model of the world. If your data is consistent with your model, then you can say that your model is possible. Of course, you should also state that other models are possible, if they, too, are consistent with the data. The models that are no longer consistent can then be changed, or our interpretation should change. Science is sometimes right only to the extent that the data proves the model—but new data can prove that model incorrect. This is how progress is made.

It is very difficult to prove something, fully and definitively. As the famous statistician George Box once said, "All models are wrong, but some are useful." We agree that all models that we create are only going to be approximations, but even as such, they can give us insights.

The same applies to nutrition science. What we know about human nutrition continues to evolve, and some past knowledge, which was scientifically proven to the best of science's ability at the time, is now being proven to be untrue. This is not because science was wrong but because science has advanced and evolved. In other cases, models can get refined—not necessarily entirely disproven, but further elucidated. Previous data, or previous limitations in our ability to develop the models, resulted in a formulation. With new data, we can sometimes revise the model and refine it so that it fits that updated data. We trust the scientific process—even when it is incomplete—because there is always room to build upon what we already know.

This brings us back to the question: Why has science never found one perfect diet that works for everyone? There have been many nutrition models that seem contradictory—vegetarian, low carb, high fat, low fat—but in fact, that seeming contradiction can be resolved if you add the individual as an active parameter to the model, including his or her genetics, microbiome, and environment. We believe that these multiple models—all claiming they work—were indeed right after all because different models have been right for different people. This is exactly what we mean by refining existing models of nutrition.

Until now, science had yet to discover the extent to which individual bodies respond differently to food. The personalized nutrition model does not disprove the previous models but shows that they are incomplete. Einstein did not disprove Newton's theories and laws but showed that they apply only in certain circumstances. Similarly, we believe that these previous nutritional models, which assumed that there exists a single diet that is best for everyone, may apply to specific study populations but are simply not consistent with the more general scientific data obtained—specifically, that different people have different responses to the same meal, demonstrating that there cannot possibly be a standardized diet that works for everyone. Instead, we propose that personalized nutrition provides a new unifying theory in nutrition science that is consistent with the emerging scientific data in its entirety.

As we set foot into this new and uncharted territory, we are excited to bring you along with us on our journey, showing you what we have learned and how models of nutrition once thought to be true have since been corrected or disproven. This is the basis for changing dietary behaviors that have had a negative influence on health in the past, and it holds the promise of changing dietary behaviors that can have a positive influence on health in the future. We have a new scientific model for you to discover, and we can show you how you can use it to personalize your diet and improve your health and life right now.

CHAPTER 4

Everything You Thought You Knew about Nutrition May Be Wrong

What if we told you that everything you thought you knew about nutrition, healthy eating, and dieting for weight loss is probably wrong? And what if we told you that even as scientists who study nutrition information, we've both been duped as well?

DR. SEGAL'S STORY

I was not always at a healthy weight. For a period of about fifteen years, I weighed 40 to 50 pounds more than I do today and had a BMI of twenty-eight to twenty-nine, which is well in the overweight category and just one to two points shy of being obese. This included my undergraduate studies in Israel, my PhD studies at Stanford, my postdoctoral work at Rockefeller, and the first few years of my faculty position at the Weizmann Institute.

You might think that I ate what I wanted and paid no attention to dietary recommendations and general knowledge, but the opposite is actually true. I was very health-conscious and even up-to-date with professional and practical wisdom, not only because I read a lot of health literature but also because my wife, who during this time became a clinical dietitian, was always health-conscious herself. She followed the commonly recommended dietary guidelines and forced them on me, whether I liked it or not!

My diet during this time was very much in line with the recommendations of the American Dietetic Association and was what many would consider quite healthy. I ate meat daily— mostly chicken. I ate primarily home-cooked foods and only occasionally at cafeterias. I rarely drank sugary drinks and was quite a heavy consumer of diet soda drinks. I did not overeat and generally ate according to my appetite. I ate vegetables, and I ate lots of low-fat foods, including low-fat yogurts and low-fat dairy products. I ate some sweets but not very often (rarely more than once a day and in measured quantities). I paid attention to calories and limited high-calorie and high-fat foods, including nuts and avocado. I limited my consumption of high-cholesterol foods like eggs and liver, I ate two to three servings of fruit daily, and I paid attention to the salt in foods and tried to limit salt intake. I did far less physical exercise than I do now, but I did some, probably one or two physical activities a week, such as basketball with friends. On paper, I was pretty much the picture of healthy living.

The reality was quite different. Despite this seemingly

health-conscious life, being overweight bothered me, and on quite a few occasions, I tried to do something about it. I went on several diets, some of them planned out in detail by my dietitian wife. Most of these diets were based on calorie restriction but used different strategies. Some limited fat intake to a minimum. I also tried various detox diets like a five-day juice-only diet. Some diets worked, some did not, but even if I lost weight, I always regained it.

DR. ELINAV'S STORY

As for me, I've battled my family history of overweight for most of my life. I've gone from one diet to another, and occasionally the diets I tried were successful, but most often they involved severe restriction in calories. This usually resulted in a sharp reduction in my weight, but it wasn't sustainable with my lifestyle, so I could never maintain these restrictive diets for very long. Over the course of a few months, I would relax the rules a little more and a little more, and eventually I would gain back everything I had lost, and then some.

When I wasn't on a diet, I would often try to adhere to the "gold standard" recommendations we all learn about: eat less fat, eat more fruits and vegetables, cut back on sugar, and so on. But I never felt like these dietary rules were quite right for me, so eventually, I relapsed into my old way of eating.

When Dr. Segal and I started calibrating the Personalized Nutrition Project to be sure our algorithms were working correctly, I happily volunteered to be one of the first "guinea pigs." I was overweight at the time, so I figured it couldn't hurt, and maybe I would learn something new. As I expected, my blood sugar levels, even during fasting (first thing in the morning), were in the "high normal" range of around 100 mg/dL. (We will tell you more about what ranges are considered normal, prediabetic, and diabetic in Chapter 6.) Then I did a trial week, eating what I would normally eat while testing, as well as experimenting with foods I had always believed to be "healthy," including bread, sushi, and fruits and vegetables of all sorts. I also tried foods that I have attempted to avoid for many years—butter on bread, ice cream, beer, and baked potatoes. I was very curious to see how I would react to this wide range of foods.

At the end of the week, I was amazed to find that bread spiked my blood sugar to frightening levels! The same was true for several other foods, some of which were an integral part of my diet, including potatoes, peppers, and even saccharin, which I used for many years as a sugar replacement in my coffee (I am an excessive coffee drinker). At the time, I also drank about 1.5 liters of diet soda every day. I was also surprised to learn what *didn't* spike my blood sugar: adding butter to my bread! When I ate ice cream and sushi and drank beer in moderation (no more than one or two beers in a day), my blood sugar levels hardly changed.

Being a skeptical scientist, I repeated my checks for these foods repeatedly, and the results remained consistent. Since then, and since we have reached the conclusion of the Personalized Nutrition Project, I have personalized my diet. I no longer eat bread and I do not consume saccharin, but I allow myself some ice cream and beer on occasion. For the last three years— the longest period I can remember—I've been able to control my blood sugar levels and weight without having to give up some of my favorite indulgences! It is my hope that our ongoing long-term studies will provide hard statistical proof that the changes I have made have indeed been the reason for my improved health measures and reduced weight—and that others can enjoy the same benefits.

HOW NUTRITION MYTHS GOT STARTED

Of course, we are not the only ones who have in the past assumed that standard nutritional information is true and accurate for everyone. There are basic nutritional rules we have all been taught since we were very young, and they are so ingrained in us that it feels wrong to question them. Imagine a roomful of children, listening to a smiling, friendly teacher who holds up a poster showing a simple but colorful pyramid or plate graphic filled with cartoonlike images of foods. Most of the pictures are foods the children recognize: bowls of spaghetti, cereal, and rice. There are loaves of bread and sheets of crackers. Carrots and lettuce, apples and grapes, a glass of milk, a slice of cheese, a turkey, a steak, a fish—pictures representing the foods the poster says people should eat to be strong and healthy. The lecture probably went something like this: "Eat most of what you see at the bottom of the pyramid [grains] and least of what you see at the top [dietary fat and added sugar]."[1] The message was clear: We should all eat up our grains and cut the fat and sugar. The stuff in the middle (vegetables, fruits, meat, and dairy products) is good to eat in moderation, or so we were told.

This seemingly benign school lesson is where nutritional

programming began for most in the United States, and it was driven home by the fact that this advice came from the U.S. government. Although some got the pre-food-pyramid lecture that showed the "five food groups" and some got the post-food-pyramid lecture showing the MyPlate graphic without the food cartoons, the advice has remained pretty much the same for many years. And because that advice came from the government, most people believed it had to be based on nutrition science and, if followed, would result in good health. No matter where or how you ate—lots of home-cooked meals or lots of fast food and processed food—the lesson was still there: Eat mostly grains like bread and pasta, then lots of fruits and vegetables, and a little less cheese and meat, and just a tiny bit of added dietary fat and sugar. This is the best way for everyone to eat.

Many other countries also adapted these U.S. guidelines (although the United States did in fact borrow the food pyramid concept from Sweden). Even the Ministry of Health of our own country of Israel used the U.S. guidelines. There is no question that the influence of these basic nutritional concepts has been widespread and international. But is the advice good? And perhaps more to the point, is it based in science?

It *sounds* like good advice, doesn't it? And it runs deep. Many people strongly believe, no matter what they hear to the contrary, that grains are good and fat is bad. Even if we read about research that suggests otherwise, and try to eat accordingly (e.g., if we try a low-carb or Paleo-style diet), it feels wrong to many people because the opposite message has been imprinted on us for most of our lives. Even when the results of such a low-carb, higher-fat diet are good, with weight loss and better health measures like blood sugar and cholesterol, there is often that lingering doubt.

That little voice inside says, *Am I hurting my health? Fat is bad. Whole grains are good.* The most avid low-carb person may occasionally wonder if all that bacon and all those bunless burgers are really doing damage. The strict low-fat vegan, even in the face of contradictory evidence such as lagging energy or high blood sugar, may feel an inner sense of security that his or her diet is best for health. Because everyone knows that low fat is best.

But is it?

Unfortunately, the real answer (like many answers in life) is a complex one. To start testing the personalization concept, the first very important thing we need to do is stop assuming we know anything about what is universally good or bad. Only when we suspend our judgment that fat or sugar or grains or even vegetables are good or bad can we discover the truth. With all these preconceptions put aside, let's now review the dietary guidelines that form the basis of our nutritional habits of our lives in the past decades, to check whether they are based on good and hard science.

As it turns out, they're not based on very good or hard science at all.

Specifically, in the formation of the dietary guidelines for Americans, there were not and still are not any randomized controlled studies that compare this government-approved dietary advice to any other diets, or that rigorously evaluate the impact of these recommendations on disease incidence and disease risk factors. Such research might result in more definitive answers, but until we have it, we cannot say that the governmental dietary guidelines for health are supportive of good health in everyone. They may benefit some people. They may not benefit some people. They may actually harm some people. Should everyone eat the recommended servings of grains? Should everyone eat the recommended servings of meat, or dairy products? Do all people need to limit sugar and added oil to the extent the guidelines recommend? Should everyone eat that much fruit, or that many vegetables, every day? Should they eat what is recommended, but in different quantities? More vegetables? Less fruit? More or less fat or protein or grain? We just don't know because we don't have the proof for or against any of these scenarios. So why have we been indoctrinated into this thinking, as if it were the law?

Steven A.

As a practicing family physician and a prediabetic, I've always followed and recommended to my patients the American Heart Association diet. I live in a small town, and more than 50 percent of my patients suffer from symptoms of the metabolic syndrome, including obesity, blood sugar disturbances, and elevated cholesterol. I have rarely seen any positive long-term responses from the diets I prescribed, but this was the diet I was told was best, and I was just passing along that information.

For many years, I blamed myself for my patients' poor compliance to my dietary recommendations. Then, when I realized I needed to lose weight and tried those same dietary recommendations I had been recommending to my patients, I realized what the problem was. Not only did I fail to see improvement in my health and weight, but I also found it extremely hard to stick to the "rules."

When I read an article about the Personalized Nutrition Project, I was intrigued. My colleagues were talking about it, and I wondered if it might be useful information for my patients as well as for my own personal struggle. I found out the project required blood sugar testing, so I decided to try it on my own. I purchased a cheap glucose sensor at my local discount store and started testing my responses to different foods. I was shocked to see how little I knew about my own body! The hearty (and heart-healthy, or so I thought) minestrone soup I loved spiked my sugar levels, but the bread that I often enjoyed with it did not. I would have guessed it would be exactly the opposite! Also, oranges made my sugar jump to the roof, but apples did not!

I couldn't help but wonder: Are we that blind to such a basic and fundamental aspect of health that we would all respond differently to different foods? I congratulate the scientists on this important discovery and hope that soon this personalized approach will be widely available to all people. When it is, I will certainly prescribe it to my patients here in the United States.

If the government's dietary recommendations aren't based on science, where did they come from? Some of the concepts arose from science that was less than rigorous, funded by the food industry, or simply limited in scope and not dependably applicable (in many of the ways we discussed in the previous chapter). Also, the group of people designing the recommendations included food industry representatives whose business and bottom line depended on people buying and eating certain foods. Of course, they would lobby for their own foods being more prominently included in the guidelines because, as we have already discussed, money is a powerful creator of bias. It is beyond the scope of this book to go into the vast and complex history of how and why different categories of foods have fallen in and out of favor, but you can read much more about the topic in books such as *Good Calories, Bad Calories* by Gary Taubes; *Food Politics* by Marion Nestle; and *Death by Food Pyramid* by Denise Minger.

All we really need to know is that we must look beyond food politics with its confusing smoke screens and misinformation, to how people really eat and how healthy they are. If you do this, you will see an incredible range of diets that produce healthy people. There are extremes: Some African people eat mostly starch, while some Inuit people eat mostly fat. There are also many more moderate examples, from cultures all over the world. Some seem to be successful. The French consume a lot of dietary fat but have very low heart disease rates. Some are less successful. In Finland, for example, people also consume a lot of dietary fat but have one of the highest heart disease rates.

Rachel K.

I was diagnosed with diabetes a few years ago. My dietitian instructed me to eat only certain types of complex carbohydrates. After taking part in the Weizmann study, I found out that whole-grain brown rice, which was recommended to me by my dietitian, spiked my blood sugar levels almost every time I ate it. This was quite a shock to me, and it made me question the rest of the recommendations I'd been given. I became much more aware of the foods I ate and decided to use foods that do not spike my glucose levels. This made a big difference for me. I was able to get better control of my blood sugar levels and was eventually able to significantly reduce the amount of diabetes medication I was taking. Thank you for enlightening me!

The truth is that so far, no diet has come out on top as universally best for everyone. Some will tell you that the Mediterranean diet, the Paleo diet, the Asian diet, or the vegan diet are best, and there are individual research projects showing that all of these have benefits. However, personalization has never been studied with these diets, and while they obviously have benefits for some (even for many), none of them will work for everyone.

We do know that when people from countries with more traditional food cultures move to countries where the Western diet is prevalent, they often gain weight and have more health issues.[2,3,4] As food writer Michael Pollan famously wrote in his book *In Defense of Food*, "the human animal is adapted to, and apparently can thrive on, an extraordinary range of different diets, but the Western diet, however you define it, does not seem to be one of them." Research shows that the U.S. diet in particular seems to be the worst manifestation of the "Western diet," especially in terms of obesity.[5] But we think this is probably because the U.S. diet, as we know it today, was born out of politics and profit rather than traditional food availability or science.

If only we were all inherently suspicious about any health advice that wasn't accompanied by comprehensive scientific references, the food pyramid and its successors, and any widely promoted dietary guideline, wouldn't be so insidious. However, research shows that people tend to follow published dietary advice, especially when it comes from the federal government.

For example, back in 2012, the American Heart Association and the American Diabetes Association jointly suggested that people should drink diet soda instead of sugar-sweetened soda for weight loss and health. As you can see from the following figure, diet soda production (we infer consumption from this statistic) has steadily risen, even though research (including some of our own) now clearly suggests that in many people, artificial sweeteners have a negative effect on both weight loss and health.[6,7]

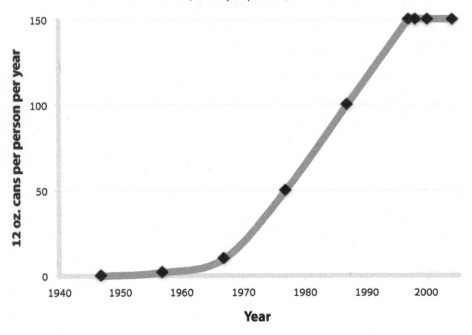

Annual diet soda drink production in the United States
(12 oz. per person)

To use another example, in 1977, when the government suggested that fat was bad and grains were good, people reduced their fat intake and increased their grain intake. Just when this happened, between 1971 and 2006, the prevalence of obesity increased from 11.9 percent to 33.4 percent in men and from 16.6 percent to 36.5 percent in women. The percentage of energy (calories) from carbohydrates increased from 44 percent to 48.7 percent, the percentage of energy from fat decreased from 36.6 percent to 33.7 percent, and the percentage of energy from protein decreased from 16.5 percent to 15.7 percent. These may seem like small changes, but these are daily averages, which can accumulate to large differences over months or years. For example, 5 percent more calories from carbs per day for someone eating a 2,000-calorie-per-day diet equals more than 100 additional carb-based calories per day, or 3,000 additional carb-based calories per month, or 36,000 additional carb-based calories per year! Trends were identical across normal-weight, overweight, and obese groups, and total energy intake (calories) increased substantially in all three BMI groups—normal weight, overweight, and obese.[8]

People believe in all kinds of things that aren't backed by science or cannot be definitively proven by science—ghosts, alien encounters, Bigfoot, a host of holistic "cures" for serious diseases... and universal food rules! Many of these beliefs can be psychologically beneficial, entertaining, or at least harmless, and some beliefs not backed by science may even be true but are as yet

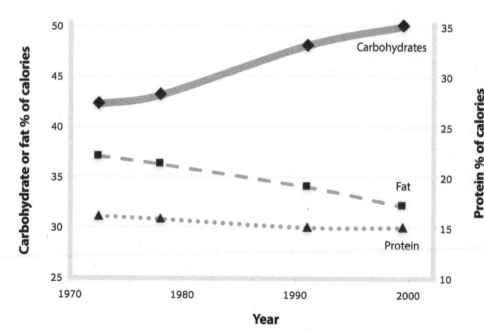

Changes in macronutrient intake in adult men aged 20–39

unproven (there may be aliens out there somewhere...who are we to say for sure?). There is still plenty for science to do, and many things science hasn't yet discovered or proven. However, when the majority of people believe something that is *not* backed by science, such as a particular dietary dogma, and when those beliefs are contradicted by science (e.g., that sugar is harmless or that artificial sweeteners are a good way to lose weight) or at least that science throws into question (e.g., that high-fat diets cause heart disease), and those beliefs have a profound influence on their health and longevity, then that is a problem—even a public health threat.

In the same way but on a smaller scale, when any individual decides to follow some bit of health advice they've read or heard about without knowing whether it is true (or true for them), then over a prolonged period of following such advice they may put their own health at risk. The diet you are currently following or the foods you are currently eating may be bad for you without your knowing it. You could be contributing to your own disease risk and obesity with the very foods you think are helping to do just the opposite.

That, unfortunately, is what has happened with nutrition—people read something, believe it, and follow it without proof that it is true or true for them. They spread the word, and others believe it, and soon everybody is juice-fasting or avoiding fruit or eliminating gluten, and all the while, there is no proven truth behind it. It is our view that making dietary changes based on unproven information has been one of the major contributors to the increase we see in metabolic diseases in the past decades.

So, before we can construct a new nutrition paradigm, we must begin to dismantle the old one by running through some commonly held beliefs about nutrition and showing you how and why they are not based in science or have been shown to be wrong.

Common Belief #1: A Calorie Is a Calorie

Technically, the term *calorie*, often used in dietary planning, actually refers to a kilocalorie, the amount of energy needed to raise the temperature of 1 kilogram of water 1 degree Celsius. The old-fashioned method for determining the calories of food was to burn the food in a sealed environment immersed in water and measure how much the temperature of the water went up. Now, calorie contents of foods are determined by professionals (or through computer programs) by using the known calories for a gram of protein (4), carbohydrates (4), and fat (9), and looking at the macronutrient content of various foods (the amount of protein, carbohydrates, and fat in a given amount of food)—then doing the math. When you look up the calorie content of food in a calorie guide or on a calorie-counting website or phone app, this is how they get those numbers.

Counting calories is common in many approaches to weight loss and operates on the idea that if you eat 100 calories and then burn 100 calories, you will "come out even" and not gain weight. However, the objective assessment of calories in a serving of any given food is quite different from the way an individual human body will digest and utilize those calories. While the old adage "calories in, calories out" is still used as a weight-loss method (we are always surprised when we see that it is still repeated so often), science has debunked this oversimplified notion that all calories operate the same in the human body.

For example, one randomized clinical trial showed that people achieved the same weight loss and similar improvements in many aspects of metabolic syndrome (like blood sugar and cholesterol levels) when they were on either a high-fat diet or a high-carb diet. However, what was most interesting about this study was that the people on the high-fat diet ate *significantly more calories* than the people on the low-fat diet.[9] If a calorie is always a calorie no matter the food source, then the people on the low-fat diet should have lost more weight, but they did not. This is just one of many studies that have called into question the notion of calorie counting solely for weight loss.

People process foods differently, extracting varying amounts of energy from the same foods. This happens for many reasons—an individual's health, age, weight, amount of fat and lean muscle, as well as how well any one person's digestive system is working, including what digestive enzymes are being effectively produced. Different people have different amounts of energy available for digestion, and efficiency varies with different people. A calorie counter could never account for all these individual variables.

Microbiome composition also affects how well energy is extracted, and because each of us has a unique microbiome environment (see Chapter 5), it makes sense that we would all extract energy differently. For example, we know that the capacity of the microbiome of obese people for extracting energy from food has been demonstrated to be enhanced compared to the microbiomes of lean people. Obese people get more energy (calories) out of a food than a lean person (this has been demonstrated in mice[10]). Calories are an aspect of the story—eating large amounts of food (lots of calories) at every meal, beyond what the body requires for energy, is likely to lead to weight gain over time. But a single large meal is not going to cause actual lasting weight gain in most people, and calories are not the only factor in weight gain, weight loss, or health.

Nutrition: What You Need

Nutrition is complex—if it weren't, we would all know what to eat and that would be the end of it. However, there are some things we know that everyone needs. No matter what diet you are on, it should contain the following:

- Fat—to assist with vitamin absorption and provide energy. In the absence of blood glucose, your body can also work just a little bit harder to get energy from fat.
- Salt—to maintain the electrolyte balance in the blood.
- Protein—for growth and repair of cells and muscles.
- Fiber—to keep the digestive system running smoothly.
- Vitamins and minerals—to assist in performing hundreds of functions in the body, like repairing cellular damage, building bone, and assisting with organ function.

You may be surprised that carbohydrates are not specifically listed. While your body can easily convert carbohydrates into glucose for energy, it is not strictly necessary. Some cultures and many individuals live primarily on fat and protein, with very few or no carbohydrates. While this way of eating is harder to comply with and follow (and probably not necessary unless you are trying to survive in an environment without any available carbohydrates), it is certainly physiologically possible.

Common Belief #2: All Fat Is Bad

Fat being bad may be the nutritional myth that is the most wide-spread and has had the most negative effect on human health in recent years: The thinking goes, if you eat a lot of fat, you will get fat. However, this is simply not true...or not *always* true. When calories stay about the same, science has demonstrated that a higher proportion of fat is more likely to *induce* weight loss than a higher proportion of carbohydrates. Again, this isn't always true in every case, but overall, *on average*, fat comes up as the weight-loss winner.

The recent low-carb and Paleo diet fads have started to change many people's minds about fat (or at least turned them against carbs). Still, most people in the mainstream believe that eating too much fat contributes to weight gain and increases the risk of diseases, especially heart disease. The American Heart Association says so. Dietitians tell their clients this. Supermarkets highlight this concept, and food companies take pride in their zero-fat products. Most people drink low-fat or nonfat milk instead of whole milk (if they drink milk at all), and if you asked the average person on the street whether a fatty prime rib or a quinoa salad was better for their health, most of them would probably choose the quinoa salad, even if they would rather eat the prime rib. This constant cultural conditioning reinforces our long-held belief: Fat is bad.

This belief is so deeply entrenched in our culture that when people read evidence to the contrary (and there is much evidence to the contrary), they have a hard time believing it. It doesn't *feel true*. They feel that they *know* fat is bad because this is the message they have been hearing for so many years, ever since childhood. They have been indoctrinated, and this conditioning is hard to break. Even some people who have embraced low-carb lifestyles admit to feeling anxious over following the diet. Is it *really* okay to eat all that meat and butter? At some point, won't we all have to pay the price?

Here's the truth: It is inaccurate to say that all fat is bad. It is an oversimplification and has not been definitively proven. There are some research studies that seem to say fat is bad, but if you read them, you will see that they often include other factors, like high calories or high sugars, and do not sufficiently isolate the fat component. Much research on fat is done on mice and rats and may or may not be reliably extrapolated to humans. A recent review of mice studies using high-fat diets—studies that were published in respected scientific journals in 2007—showed that those studies were not accurately portrayed because the high-fat diets they used consisted of 60 percent lard, 20 percent sucrose, and 20 percent milk protein—essentially mouse junk food that was also very high in sugar and protein.[11] Saying that fat caused the cognitive problems or obesity or other health issues in the mice ignores the fact that it could just as well have been the sucrose or the milk protein. In addition, the control mice in these studies were being fed a standard mouse chow full of soy protein, so the plant estrogens in that soy food could have also skewed the control results. Even more important, these were not good controls because to really isolate the fat, the control diet would have to be identical to the "high-fat" diet except for the fat content. The other parts of the diets were not the same, making the results even more suspect. This is an example of faulty science that does not sufficiently isolate the tested component. There were too many confounding factors to draw any reliable conclusions about fat. But as kids learning about nutrition in school, or even as adults reading generalized dietary advice, we are not introduced to the many intricacies and limitations of studies like these. We are just "sold" the simple take-home message that fat is bad.

To complicate matters even further, there are many types of fat. It doesn't make sense to say, "fat is bad" or "low fat is good" if you don't specify what type of fat you are talking about. The fat in bacon is not the same as the fat in a bottle of canola oil or in a French fry or in a drizzle of cold-pressed olive oil or in a coconut, neither literally nor biochemically.

For example, there is good evidence that artificial trans fats (an industrial process that makes liquid fats into solid fats) are detrimental to health.[12] But for other types of fats—for example, those higher in saturated, monounsaturated, or polyunsaturated fatty acids, such as steak, olive oil, or nuts and seeds, respectively—the results are quite mixed. Research shows that different kinds of natural fats have different associations with disease risk.[13,14] One study showed unfavorable metabolic effects (like obesity and insulin resistance) in rats fed extra lard or olive oil (mainly long-chain saturated fatty acids and monounsaturated fatty acids), but they did not see the negative impact in rats fed with coconut oil and fish oil (mostly polyunsaturated vegetable fats or medium-chain saturated fatty acids).[15] Another study demonstrated that there was no evidence that saturated fat was associated with death from any cause during the course of the study or with cardiovascular disease, ischemic stroke, or type 2 diabetes, but industrial trans fat was associated with all of these[16] (the Food and Drug Administration [FDA] now limits trans fats in foods).

Fat-centric diets also have varying effects, and there is even plenty of research that suggests these diets have good rather than bad effects. Many studies comparing low-carb (assumed to be high fat) and low-fat (assumed to be high carb) diets in humans for weight loss or heart disease risk effects showed that the low-carb diets were *just as* effective as the low-fat diets, or slightly more effective, or much more effective, depending on the study you read.[17] There is also very little good evidence that high-fat diets are linked to heart disease,[18] but there has been plenty of research showing that low-carbohydrate and Mediterranean diets (both typically higher in fat) can be more effective for weight loss and improved insulin sensitivity and fasting glucose, in general.[19]

When looking at these trends, it's helpful to look at meta-analyses, which are studies that analyze the results from other multiple studies to draw a broad-based conclusion. Because meta-analyses are based on very large numbers with very long periods of follow-up, they offer good overviews as compared to single studies. Good examples of long-term studies that are frequently cited in research are the Nurses' Health Study[20] and the Framingham Heart Study[21] because they contained so much broad information collected over a long period of time from many people. Many of these studies have shown that low-carb diets that are higher in fat content achieve greater weight-loss results than low-fat diets and improve risk factors for heart disease, including raising HDL cholesterol (the kind known to reduce heart disease risk), lowering triglycerides (high levels of which may be associated with heart disease risk), and reducing heart disease.[22,23]

Epidemiologically, researchers have not found a reliable

association between the consumption of dietary fat and the incidence of heart disease. So, as you can see, fat may not be that bad. You must take advice from influential organizations like the American Heart Association that tell you to eat less fat with a grain of salt (and we'll get to salt soon). To the American Heart Association's credit, they recently revised their advice to recommend some fats and to discourage the use of saturated fat, trans fat, sodium, red meat, sweets, and sugar-sweetened beverages. They also suggest an emphasis on nontropical vegetable oils[24]— advice that is somewhat more in line with current research (although there are still many mixed results on this topic). This is an indication that attitudes are changing, slowly, as they face food industry opposition and lag far behind current scientific research.

At the same time, making any absolute proclamation about fat as it applies to everyone is also an oversimplification. Fat might be more harmful to some people than others, and there is some evidence that some kinds of fat cause inflammation, oxidative stress, insulin resistance,[25] heart disease, and cognitive decline.[26] There is also evidence that extremely low-fat diets can reverse heart disease progression for some people.[27] Then again, that doesn't mean they will work for everyone.

None of this means that "fat is always bad," nor does it mean that "fat is always good." In general, we think it is safe to say that most research shows that fat *in general* does not have a negative effect for *most* people (or mice or rats) but that *some* types of fat, especially in excess, may *sometimes* have a negative effect on *some* people (or mice or rats). That may sound a little confusing, but you will soon see why it is a smart and accurate perspective.

A Grain (or Two) of Salt

Many people feel guilty eating high-salt foods because they believe salt raises blood pressure in everyone, which increases the risk of strokes and myocardial infarctions. However, in healthy people, sodium intake has a negligible effect on blood pressure, according to a meta-analysis of fifty-eight studies on the effects of sodium on blood pressure.[28] In fact, salt is very important for proper cell function, and our bodies have extensive mechanisms for regulating sodium levels in the blood and in and around our cells. When the levels get too high, our cells excrete salt for elimination, and when they are too low, they try to intake more salt from the blood. These processes have evolved for billions of years and are at work in the complex human body. While it is likely true that some people are more sensitive to salt than others are, this is certainly not a reason to enact a global dietary rule about this essential mineral.

Common Belief #3: High-Carbohydrate / Low-Fat Diets Are Bad

Just as there are no definitive studies that show a high-fat diet is harmful for everyone, there are also no definitive studies that show a high-carb diet is harmful for everyone. First of all, most foods contain some carbohydrates—sugar, fruit, grains, starchy vegetables, even non-starchy vegetables contain carbs. It is our personal opinion that there are more studies showing the superiority of low-carb diets for weight loss and disease prevention than there are studies showing the superiority of low-fat diets, but that doesn't mean carbs are bad. It only means that a high percentage of calories from carbs are bad for weight loss and disease prevention *in some people*. Even if they hinder results in *the majority of people*, they do not have the same effect on *all people*. Every study has those participants who are not affected the way the majority is affected, and that goes for successful low-carb studies as well as low-fat studies.

And even if there are more studies showing the benefits of a low-carb-style diet, there are certainly studies that show the benefits of a low-fat diet, especially when compared to a standard American diet or other specific diets (such as "diabetes diets"). In some of these studies, high-carb diets contributed to weight loss and improved health measures in some situations and for many people. There is especially compelling evidence showing how high-carb, very-low-fat diets have reversed advanced heart disease in some people. For weight loss alone, a high-carb diet may not work as well or as quickly for many people, but it may work better for some.

And perhaps even more important to remember, there is certainly no proof that carbohydrate-rich foods, as an overall category that does not distinguish between different kinds of carbs, are harmful in any way. You could make a case that refined sugar and refined grains have detrimental health effects in many people, but it's harder to prove this when you look at whole grains, fruits, and vegetables, which also contain a lot of nutrients and fiber.

Unfortunately, there is plenty of faulty science in low-fat studies, just as there are in high-fat studies. For example, many studies on low-fat diets also include caloric restriction or reduction. Is eating low fat helping with weight loss or more positive health effects, or is it the calorie restriction? If you don't isolate

these elements, you cannot say for sure which element is causing the effect or whether it is an effect based on the combination of two elements—low fat and low calorie. But as we have
pointed out, many of the studies that compare low-fat and/or
high-carbohydrate diets to low-carb and/or high-fat diets show
fairly similar results. While some research shows that a low-fat
or a high-carbohydrate diet can be more effective for weight
loss, blood sugar stability, and heart health than a higher fat diet,
especially in people with diabetes or glucose intolerance,[29,30]
many other studies (mentioned in the previous section) show
the opposite.

When low carb came out ahead, as it did in some studies,
the difference after twelve months was about the same, and in
some cases, the low-carb dieters had elevated cholesterol levels
(especially the "bad" LDL cholesterol),[31] while those on the
high-carb / low-fat diet sometimes had reduced body weight and
improved levels for cholesterol, triglycerides, and blood pressure. Sometimes, the high-carb / low-fat dieters regained more
weight after three years, although their positive health measures
remained improved.[32]

Other studies that have shown a low-carb diet is more effective in weight loss than a high-carb / low-fat diet did not use a
truly low-fat diet. Instead, they usually limited fat to about 30
percent, which is close to the amount in the standard American
diet (which is generally considered to contain about 50 percent
calories from carbs, 15 percent from protein, and about 35 percent from fat), so the results may not be as telling as if the low-
fat diet were a truly low-fat diet. One analysis of multiple studies
showed "overwhelming evidence" that very-low-fat diets (with

fat levels below 15 percent of calories) resulted in reductions in saturated fat, dietary cholesterol, and body weight.[33] Another study showed moderate improvements in cholesterol levels when saturated fat was replaced with polyunsaturated fat, and even more dramatic improvements when all fat was drastically reduced.[34]

And what about the type of carbs? As we've already mentioned, fruit, vegetables, grains, sugar, and corn syrup are all high-carb foods, but research has demonstrated that generally eating more dietary fiber reduces the risk of obesity and diabetes,[35] while eating more sugar increases the risk of dying from heart disease,[36] and eating more refined carbs in the form of corn syrup was correlated with a higher risk of diabetes.[37] One study reviewed existing research and showed that based on observational studies, whole-grain consumption was generally associated with disease risk reduction, especially of heart disease, diabetes, and cancer, as well as weight management and digestive health, but other studies didn't necessarily demonstrate this effect.[38] There are quite a few studies demonstrating the deleterious effects of sugar consumption. While there is scant evidence that vegetables or fruit have any ill effects on human health (and we know that many of the compounds they contain are protective), there is plenty of evidence that sugar and refined grains (like white flour) have some negative effects on health, including a greater risk of dying from heart disease,[39] developing diabetes,[40,41] and feeding cancer cells. The association between sugar and cancer is an old theory that is coming back into fashion as one of the latest research focuses in cancer prevention and remission is investigating the role of blood sugar and insulin in cancer cell metabolism.[42]

As you can see, the carb picture is complex. The essential point is that, according to the scientific literature, low-carb diets that are high in fat can improve weight and health measures in many people, and low-fat diets that are high in carbs may also improve weight and health measures in others. There is evidence for both diets—which, in a sense, is evidence for neither. This all comes back to our theory: While there may be discernible trends when looking at averages, the answer to the seemingly confounding variability lies in the differences among individuals—low-carb diets may work for some; high-carb diets may work for others.

But what if all this macronutrient juggling was for nothing? In our opinion, based on our own research, it seems likely that nobody needs to be particularly low fat or low carb. Because many of these studies have been performed on small numbers of people, person-specific differences likely lead to results that are relatively random regarding which macronutrients have which effects, and which dietary strategy appears to come out ahead. One study may appear to favor outcome A, and another may appear to favor outcome B, only because everyone in each small study is reacting to the foods differently. Instead, perhaps people simply need to determine *which* carbs and *which* fats and *which* proteins work best for them.

Is Dietary Cholesterol Bad for You?

You may remember a few years ago when a publicity campaign funded by the Egg Board proclaimed that eggs were now safe to eat again. Eggs have fallen in and out of favor over the years largely due to their cholesterol content, but of course, they are not the only sources of dietary cholesterol. Most products of animal origin contain cholesterol, and plenty of doctors—especially cardiologists—spend plenty of time warning their patients to avoid dietary cholesterol, although cholesterol is an important component of the body and especially the brain.

Although many people still believe that dietary cholesterol is bad and limit their egg and animal product intake because they are worried about cholesterol, the truth is that this belief has long been debunked. There is *no evidence* that cholesterol in the diet affects levels of cholesterol in the blood. The body manufactures cholesterol and regulates cholesterol levels, and this is unrelated to eating cholesterol. There may be reasons not to eat eggs or steak or shrimp, but your serum cholesterol level is not one of them.[43]

Common Belief #4: Going on a Diet Works

In many cases, diets—whether calorie-restricted or manipulating macronutrient intake (like low carb or low fat)—work for some people in the short term. You know this if you have ever lost weight or felt better on a diet. But did that weight stay off? Did you continue to feel better? There is evidence that diets do not generally work very well at all. You might lose some, but you might gain it all back…or most of it. As you can see from the following chart, which depicts a very-low-calorie diet, a standard diet (this was nonspecific but could be any diet, such as something a dietitian would give you), and a diet plus exercise, weight loss for all methods happened initially, but for all three diets most of the weight came back. That's not very encouraging.

Most weight-loss strategies initially have a dramatic effect, but after several months, the effect levels out. For example, drastically cutting food intake (such as with a very-low-calorie diet)

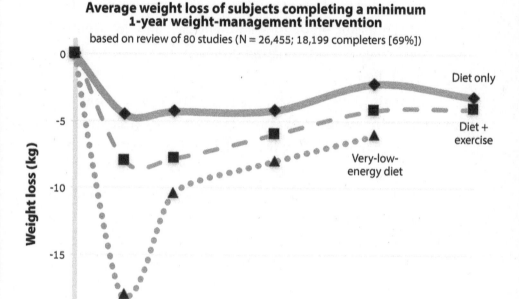

Average weight loss of subjects completing a minimum 1-year weight-management intervention

based on review of 80 studies (N = 26,455; 18,199 completers [69%])

often has the most dramatic initial effect, but in most cases, a couple of years later, the weight comes back.

Consider a recent highly publicized study on the participants in the television show *The Biggest Loser*. The participants in the study all lost large amounts of weight through exercise and calorie restriction during their time on this show, but the study showed that this weight loss induced their bodies to lower their metabolic rate and that even six years later, the participants' metabolisms were still so low that they were not able to eat the same number of calories as someone else of a similar weight who had never been overweight[44] (the study called this "persistent metabolic adaptation").

Other research shows that in many cases, dieting is a

consistent predictor of eventual weight gain, not loss;[45,46] dieting was a significant predictor of weight gain in adolescents;[47]
and binge-eating and other eating disorders increased with the
frequency of dieting.[48]

We recently came out with a study with a pretty dramatic
result. We demonstrated that the gut microbes (microbiome)
of dieters "remember" being overweight, so that even after the
weight is lost, the microbiome does not change to the microbiome of a lean person. That affects how the body responds to
food in a manner that enhances postdiet weight regain. We'll
talk about it more in the next chapter.

Another big misconception about dieting is that people don't
follow the diet. This is certainly true some of the time, but in
our experience and research, we would like to suggest that in
many cases, people follow the diets, and the diets either still
don't work or result in ultimate weight gain. Many people move
from one fashionable diet to the next, looking for that silver bul-
let diet that will finally work for them. But what really works?
That seems to depend on the person—how well they tolerate the
diet, how well they comply with the guidelines of the diet, how
long they stay on the diet, and whether the lifestyle changes they
make are effective for them or not.

Another problem is that many diets simply aren't well
defined. For example, you could eat "low carb" or "low fat" but
still eat primarily processed foods and very few foods with good
nutrient content. Or, you could eat "low carb" or "low fat" and
make excellent choices by eating nutrient-dense foods. You
could technically follow a vegetarian diet and eat macaroni
and cheese every day, or follow a vegan diet but live on vegan
cookies and French fries. Alternatively, you could be following

a vegetarian or vegan diet but choose primarily fiber-rich and protein-rich plant foods like vegetables and minimally processed whole grains, along with cold-pressed oils and organic fruit.

Along those same lines, you could technically follow a Paleo diet but live solely on cheap fatty meat and sweets made from processed coconut products, or an Atkins diet where you mostly eat bacon, bunless burgers, and cheese. Or, you could call your diet the very same thing but eat mostly nonstarchy, nutrient-dense vegetables and very small amounts of high-quality meat protein.

You can also make macronutrient assumptions about a diet that focuses on eliminating a category of foods. For example, a Paleo diet, generally considered to be "low carb," could be high in carbs if it includes a lot of fruit and starchy vegetables. A vegan diet, generally considered to be "low fat," could be high in fat if it includes a lot of vegetable oil, nuts, and fatty foods like avocadoes. It all depends on what foods you choose, so a diet by any name as a weight-loss strategy is meaningless.

Finally (and most critically), it should now be obvious that some dietary strategies work for some people and not for others. Some thrive on fat as a primary fuel source, while others don't. Some thrive on plant-based diets, while others feel better and lose more weight on diets that include fairly large amounts of animal protein. Some people don't feel the need to eat very much, while others have hearty appetites and eat more calories without gaining more weight. You can see this from the following figure, which shows the results of two separate diets tested on a group of people. The first diet didn't work at all on anyone. The second diet worked well on some but made others gain weight. There is no way to know which dietary intervention will work for you, if at all. Is it worth depriving yourself?

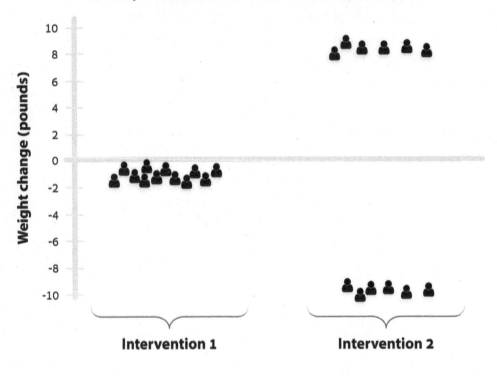

Two dietary interventions with similar average effects, but very different effects on individual participants

Tami E.

As a devoted mother of two, I've always taken the utmost effort to provide my kids with a balanced healthy diet. I spent hours looking over the Internet, consulting with my friends, and preparing lunches for my daughter, who is in second grade, and my son, who is in kindergarten. My kids are happy, healthy, and active, but like many people in our family (and many kids in her class) my eight-year-old daughter is overweight.

My husband and I assumed this was genetic, but the fact is that only the last two generations of our family have struggled with weight issues. I became concerned when I heard a national news story that childhood obesity is associated with later-life health problems, so I felt like I should do something about it. I mean, even our former First Lady, Michelle Obama, made this her platform! The problem was I didn't know what to do. My daughter was eating well, as far as the rules of nutrition go, and she was active, playing on a soccer team. It certainly didn't seem appropriate to put such a young girl on a diet.

Then I heard about personalized nutrition in a national news story, and it struck a chord. I began testing my blood sugar responses to foods using a household glucose monitor, and I was surprised to see that my responses to food were not at all what I expected. For example, coffee seems to spike my blood sugar, while oatmeal cookies do not. Bananas spike me, but tomatoes don't (I read that many people get blood sugar spikes after eating tomatoes). My previous notion of how to keep my own and my family's diets healthy sort of collapsed in front of my eyes.

Then I thought, *If healthy food isn't what I thought it was for me, it probably isn't what I think it is for the rest of my family.* I can't wait to learn how I can improve my entire family's diet using this method.

What all these nutritional misconceptions really show us is that while nutritional information is interesting, generalized nutritional rules cannot be universally effective. When solid scientific information conflicts with other solid scientific information, it is not because of the diet or the food. It is because while science seeks to find a one-size-fits-all approach to diet, it's not possible because everyone reacts differently to different foods, and there isn't a dietary strategy that will work for everyone.

But this is good news. This means that for the many people who have tried diets and failed, there is hope. It's likely the diet has not worked because it was the wrong diet for you. Food responses and *personalized nutrition* are the answers to the problem of what to eat for health and weight loss. Most diets come at the problem from the wrong perspective—foods and the nutrients in them. To solve the diet question, we need to look at the individual and examine what makes each of us have a unique response to what we eat. To do that, let's take a closer look at what is going on inside you, so you can better understand why your own food reactions must certainly be unique to you.

CHAPTER 5

The Universe Inside Your Gut—
and Why It Matters

In 1883, a fifteen-year-old girl named Mary Mallon immigrated to the United States from Ireland. After working in various households doing sundry domestic duties, she was hired as a cook in 1906 by a wealthy New York banker named Charles Henry Warren, who rented a home on Oyster Bay on the north shore of Long Island, New York. That summer and into early fall, six of the eleven household members contracted typhoid fever. At the time, typhoid fever was fatal about 10 percent of the time, so the number of people contracting the disease was very concerning.

The family hired a sanitary engineer named George Soper to investigate. At first, Soper suspected freshwater clams as the culprit, but not everyone who had fallen ill had eaten them. Finally, he uncovered the truth, and his results, which he published in 1906 in the *Journal of the American Medical Association* (*JAMA*), revealed that Mary Mallon, who had been only moderately ill with typhoid, was the first documented case in the United States of a healthy carrier of a bacterium called *Salmonella typhi*.

But Mary denied being the cause of the contagion. She had barely been sick. She was not sick when she was accused. She could not believe that she was responsible. Soper, however, was convinced. He discovered that Mary Mallon had previously served as a cook for eight different families, and seven of those families had experienced outbreaks of typhoid—resulting in twenty-two cases of illness, some of which resulted in death.

Typhoid fever was going around New York that year—some 3,000 New Yorkers were affected—and Mary Mallon may have been largely responsible for the outbreak. Without antibiotics (they would not be available until 1948), the situation was grave. Soper convinced the New York Department of Health and the police to force Mary Mallon to come in for stool sample testing, and although she ran, they finally found her and obtained the samples from her. Sure enough, the samples were positive for *Salmonella typhi*, the microbe causing typhoid fever. She was quarantined in a cottage near a hospital on North Brother Island. She tried to sue the health department but lost and was confined for two years.

The hospital tried to cure Mary. They treated her with laxatives, brewer's yeast, and a urinary antiseptic called urotropine, but nothing worked. They wanted to remove her gallbladder, because they suspected it was the source of the shedding bacteria, but she refused to consent to that surgery. During those two years, 120 out of 163 of her stool samples tested positive, but unfortunately, no one ever fully explained the situation to her, so she was adamant that she was being held captive and should be set free.

In 1910, Mary was released thanks to a new and sympathetic health commissioner, on condition that she never again work as a cook. However, Mary did not comply with this condition. She changed her name to Mary Brown and immediately got a job as a cook at Sloane Maternity in Manhattan, where in a period of just three months, she was responsible for the infection of twenty-five people, including doctors, nurses, and staff. Two people died. When she was found out, she was given the name "Typhoid Mary" and was lambasted in newspaper cartoons. She was infamous. She was also returned to quarantine on North Brother Island and remained there for the next twenty-six years, in virtual isolation, until her death in 1938.

By the time Mary Mallon died, New York health officials had discovered 400 other people who were deemed "healthy carriers" of *Salmonella typhi*, but Mary Mallon was the only one who was ever forcibly quarantined. All told, "Typhoid Mary" was responsible for the infection of 125 people and five deaths.[1]

It's a sad story, but also an instructional one: The bacteria inside your gut can have a powerful effect on your life, your health, and the health of those around you. Some can harm you. Some can harm others. Much of it is beneficial and lives in harmony with you. It is not genetically part of you. It is along for the ride. But you can tend this *microbiome* in a way that can encourage the growth of the good bacteria and discourage the growth of the bad.

Bacteria Bad Guys

Typhoid fever is much less common than it was in the early 1900s, when there were tens of thousands of cases of this virulent disease, thanks mostly to improvements in sanitation. There are fewer than 400 cases of typhoid fever reported annually in the United States, mostly in people who have traveled to less-developed parts of the world, like Mexico, South America, and India.[2]

But while typhoid may not be as much of an issue today, we have other bacterial issues to contend with. One of the most virulent and contagious is *Clostridium difficile* (*C. diff*), a bacterium that drives a serious gastrointestinal infection mainly seen in hospitalized patients and causes diarrhea, severe abdominal pain, fever, and, in some extreme cases, death. In 2011, there were 29,000 deaths from *C. diff* in the United States alone, and when people do not die from it, the hostile takeover of this bacterium can make them miserable and drastically affect quality of life. People with diseases of the colon, like Crohn's disease or other inflammatory bowel diseases; those suffering from colorectal cancer; older people; and those using certain medications, such as broad-spectrum antibiotics, are particularly at risk, but a *C. diff* infection could happen to anyone. We can treat *C. diff* infection with antibiotics, but there are cases that have become so resistant that no medications are available for treating it, and science is actively seeking better treatments for the *C. diff* problem.

WHO IS LIVING IN YOUR GUT?

Your gut is host to 40 trillion microbial cells and up to 1,000 different microbial species. In fact, the cells in your gut bacteria approximate the total number of your own cells. If you were to go by cell count alone, you would be only about half human,[3] with your measly 30 trillion human cells.[4]

These inner microbes you host include mostly bacteria, but

also viruses, fungi, parasites, and other microscopic organisms that have their own DNA, with about 200 times the number of genes that you have.[5] That adds up to approximately 25,000 human genes and approximately 5 million bacterial genes! While scientists spend a lot of time studying human genes, that's only about 1 percent of the diversity of genetic material that each of us carry. We don't yet know what most of these microbial genes do—this is an exciting new area of research. (We also still don't know what many human genes do either, but we have been studying them for a longer amount of time. We are only now beginning to study the nature and effect of the millions of bacterial genes each of us host.)

Microbes live on and inside us, wherever our bodies engage with the outside world—in our skin, mouth, gut, respiratory tract, and genitourinary system. We call this system the *microbiome*, and we all have microbiomes at each of these body sites. Yet, the microbiome was not generally recognized until the late 1990s.[6] Of all the microbiomes in our bodies, the gut's is by far the most diverse, complex, and physiologically important. In contrast, the insides of our bodies (our blood system and internal organs) are generally devoid of microbes, or at least large numbers of them, and are generally considered sterile—unless microbes enter into them through a wound or an infection.

The Species in Your Feces

Recent advances in DNA sequencing have allowed us to start studying the microbiome. The source of the genetic material to analyze the bacteria in someone's microbiome is a stool sample because a large part of the solid content of feces is bacteria. The bacteria in your microbiome reproduce, grow, and die through-out your life. On any given day, 10 percent of your gut microbes are shed and the body removes them via feces, so studying the feces is a good way to get access to the genetic material of the bacteria and can aid in determining the microbiome content in your gut at any given moment.

Typical feces composition is approximately 75 percent water and 25 percent solid matter, including:

- undigested fiber and solidified components of digestive juices (30 percent);
- bacteria (30 percent), both helpful and harmful;
- fat (10 to 20 percent);
- inorganic matter (10 to 20 percent); and
- protein (2 to 3 percent).

The Discovery of the Microbiome

The first scientific evidence that microorganisms are part of the human system emerged in the mid-1880s, when Austrian pedi-atrician Theodor Escherich observed a type of bacteria (later named *Escherichia coli*, or *E. coli*) in the intestinal flora of healthy children as well as in children affected by diarrheal disease.

An early microbiome aficionado was Élie Metchnikoff, a prominent Nobel laureate and one of the founding fathers of modern immunology. One day in the late nineteenth century, he looked in his primitive light microscope at a fresh stool sam-ple and was amazed to see that it was crawling with countless live bacteria. He realized that this "world within a world" could be fundamentally important for our lives. He started drinking a glass of sour milk every day, believing that it might change his gut microbes for the better, and he even published a work called "Prolongation of Life—Optimistic Studies," in which he postulated that these microbes might enable us to prolong our lives. At the time, there was no method available to study the microbes Metchnikoff had observed. The field of microbiology was busy focusing on fighting the "bad" disease-causing bacteria, and the microbiome would not be generally recognized as an important part of human bodies or health for almost a century, in the late 1990s.

It has been only about ten years since scientists have been able to study these bacteria extensively, using advanced genetic techniques. Many of these bacteria are "spoiled," in that they require very specific conditions to thrive and grow and cannot therefore live outside of the human body. Some, for example, are obligate anaerobes, meaning they are microorganisms that are killed by normal atmospheric concentrations of oxygen. We didn't know how to grow them outside the body for study. Around 2006 to 2007, advances in DNA sequencing allowed us to determine the entire gut content from a stool sample and sequence it, thereby identifying the collection of microbes within and circumventing the need to culture the microorganisms for study. This has resulted in making the microbiome one of the most exciting new areas of research. There has been an explosion of new research on the microbiome lately (see the following figure), and we ourselves are not immune to the excitement. As you will see in this chapter, we have made discoveries and published research on several key areas that are influenced by the microbiome in ways that may surprise you. But we aren't the only ones studying this

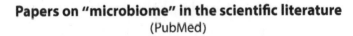

Papers on "microbiome" in the scientific literature
(PubMed)

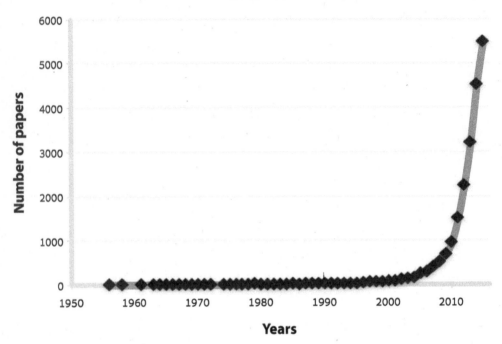

active, growing field of research. Many scientists are now study-ing the microbiome's many aspects, qualities, functions, and influences.

The most exciting area of research is that we are beginning to uncover causative aspects of the microbiome, rather than simply its associations to many common diseases. In other words, we are learning what directly influences the microbiome and what the microbiome can cause to happen, rather than only knowing that certain conditions and certain microbes exist simultaneously. We are making similar advances in human genetics—learning causative aspects rather than just associative aspects—but the exciting difference between genetics and the microbiome is that while we can't change our genes, we can alter our microbiome. We are discovering how we can therapeutically modulate a key element of human health.

What Your Gut Microbiome Does for You

Although it may sound off-putting to think that your body is full of bacteria, rest assured that you live in a symbiotic relationship with bacteria, and those microbes do a lot to improve your life. For example, your microbiome provides the following:

- **Energy:** Approximately 10 to 20 percent of our energy is supplied not by our body's breakdown of food but by bacterial breakdown of food. Your microbiome produces digestive enzymes and vitamins the body needs. It also helps determine how and how much energy you extract from the food you eat.[7,8]
- **Essential vitamins:** Your microbiome produces essential vitamins that your body requires and cannot produce on its own, like vitamin K (menaquinone), vitamin B_{12} (cobalamin), vitamin B_9 (folate), and vitamin B_2 (riboflavin).[9]

    Vitamin B_{12} is especially important for maintaining healthy nerve cells and assisting in the production of DNA and RNA (the body's genetic material). Vitamin B_{12} in food comes almost exclusively from animal products, especially shellfish, crustaceans, and beef, but vegetarians may not be deficient in vitamin B_{12} if they have a healthy microbiome, especially containing lots of *Bifidobacterium* and *Lactobacillus*. The most famous B_{12} producer is

Lactobacillus reuteri, a common bacterium in the human intestines and part of your microbiome.[10]

Vitamin B$_9$, or folate, is also extremely important. Usually it is found in fresh, uncooked, unfrozen vegetables, but like B$_{12}$, folate can be produced by lactic acid bacteria like *Lactobacillus* and *Bifidobacterium*[11] in your gut.

- **Immunity:** Your microbiome helps to regulate your immune system,[12] and in fact, important features of a healthy immune system require the microbiome in order to develop properly. Your microbiome assists in recognizing invaders and helps the body not attack itself (as it does in an autoimmune disease). The microbiome also helps create a barrier against pathogens and may determine which allergies you get and what allergens won't affect you.[13]

- **Health:** Our microbiome also determines, for better or for worse, our health status. In the past ten years, our understanding of associations between the microbiome and health has expanded greatly, and we have discovered microbiome associations with a broad range of conditions, including obesity;[14,15] asthma, allergies, and autoimmune conditions;[16,17,18,19,20,21,22] depression[23,24] and other mental illnesses;[25,26] inflammatory bowel disease, including Crohn's disease and ulcerative colitis; neurodegeneration;[27,28,29] cancer; and vascular disease.[30,31] There is much research to be done on how we might manipulate the microbiome to get better control over these many conditions.

- **Infant health.** Bacteria in the microbiome of the mother, called *oligosaccharides*, are delivered to the infant through breast milk and help to shape the infant microbiome in

Human microbiome and conditions that were associated with disruption in microbiome composition and function

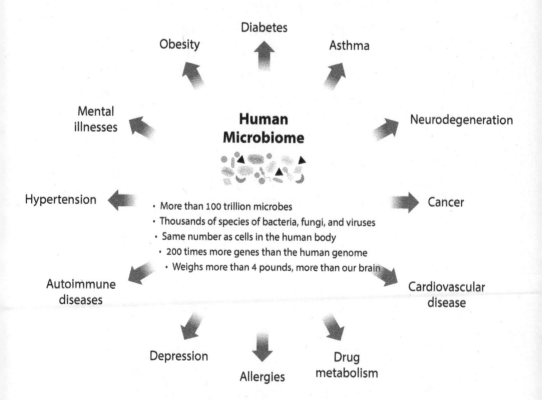

- More than 100 trillion microbes
- Thousands of species of bacteria, fungi, and viruses
- Same number as cells in the human body
- 200 times more genes than the human genome
- Weighs more than 4 pounds, more than our brain

a healthy way[32]—a possible argument in favor of breast-feeding. Microbes may also pass from mom to infant as the child moves through the birth canal (this is currently an active area of research). We think it's quite amazing to see evolution in action in this way, as substances from the mother are literally shaping the microbiome of the next generation. This is just one more demonstration of the importance of the microbiome in our development and an example of the coevolution of humans and bacteria. We have evolved along with our microbiomes and at this point, we need them to survive (just as they need us to survive).

Saleyha A.

I always felt that food had a different effect on me than it did on my sisters. We all ate the same foods every evening at dinner, and yet I was always chubby and they were always slim. If I wanted to be like them, I believed, I would have to cut out bread and rice and pasta from my diet. Carbs were bad. That was the latest dietary wisdom.

I also noticed that every time I ate, I was tired. I'm not just talking about an energy slump. I'm talking, *I need to lie down and sleep right this minute.* I thought maybe I was just lazy, but I didn't understand how other people would eat the same foods I was eating and be wide awake. I heard a theory that "all blood rushes to the stomach after eating, to digest the food," so I decided that was what I was feeling.

When I was a junior doctor, I couldn't afford this extreme postmeal energy slump, so I just quit eating lunch when I was on the wards. But by late afternoon, I was starving, and I would eat chocolates or biscuits left at the nursing station by grateful patients. Of course, this made me even sleepier. Those "sugar lows" came on quickly, and the only way I could find to combat them was to eat even more sugar, to keep me "charged" through the rest of the workday. At home, I lived on grapes, tomatoes, salads, and tuna. I never ate bread, and when I dared to eat ice cream, I felt so guilty that it usually wasn't worth it.

When my producer on our BBC show, *Trust Me, I'm a Doctor,* asked me if I wanted to participate in the Personalized Nutrition Project and report on it, I was keen but also didn't expect to learn much. I thought that by the age of forty-four, I had a pretty good idea already of how my body responded to food.

I could not have been more wrong. My gut bacteria profile and blood sugar testing revealed that both grapes and tomatoes gave me huge blood sugar spikes, while ice cream actually did not. Most surprising to me was that toast with butter did not spike my blood sugar even a little bit.

I've since adopted a different style of eating, based on what I learned from participating in the study, and it has changed me. My skin looks better, I have energy all day long, including after meals and in the late afternoon, and best of all, I've dropped a lot of weight, and I'm still losing, without even feeling like I am eating any less than before. I feel great, and I believe this experience has been a significant turning point in my health and my life.

When a Good Microbiome Goes Bad

Every microbiome contains a wide range of different kinds of bacteria, and some of it can cause problems, especially when conditions are suitable for the more pathogenic bacteria to thrive. If your microbiome gets out of balance, some of the following can occur:

- **Aging.** The microbiome has been linked with aging, especially when it becomes less diverse.[33] A diverse microbiome is a vigorous and more effective microbiome, but a loss of bacterial diversity (fewer different species) has been associated with both physical frailty and reduced cognitive performance (as with dementia). We mainly observe this in people who live in developed countries where microbiomes have become less diverse, probably due to Western diets that are also less diverse, higher in sugar, and lower in fiber. Research[34,35] in mice shows that eating diets over three or four generations that are more Western and have less fiber leads to the extinction of specific microbes that cannot be restored when a high-fiber diet is resumed. Fiber is not digested by human digestive enzymes and goes directly to the gut bacteria in the intestines, where it serves as a food source for bacteria. Restoring the lost bacterial species requires adding the missing bacteria (as is done through intensive probiotic therapy, which may or may not be effective) and/or shifting the diet toward more diverse food ingredients found in traditional foods, meaning natural, unprocessed foods that could reintroduce some of the lost bacteria and also provide more fiber to support a larger and more diverse bacterial population.

- **More metabolic syndrome (or less).** The microbiome has been most heavily studied in relation to obesity, diabetes, hypercholesterolemia, and fatty liver, which often co-occur together in the same person and, when this happens, are called "the metabolic syndrome." These are very common diseases throughout the world that constitute a serious epidemic that has developed in the last century. They also predispose people to many dangerous complications, including heart attacks, stroke, clogging of arteries, kidney disease, and more. We'll elaborate more on the metabolic syndrome in Chapter 6 when we discuss the importance of a normal blood sugar level. Many factors contribute to the metabolic syndrome epidemic, and many of these may be linked to changes in our modern gut microbiome. The microbiome may, in fact, not only be associated with the metabolic syndrome but may contribute to many of the manifestations associated with the metabolic syndrome, including obesity, diabetes, and hypercholesterolemia. The microbiome influences our metabolism by altering our immune system, modulating our hormonal system, changing the repertoire of small molecules (metabolites) secreted from our gut into our bloodstream,[36] and even affecting our nervous system. For example, research in rodents shows that increased production of a specific metabolite called *acetate* activates an arm of our peripheral nervous system, termed the *parasympathetic nervous system*, which in turn increases glucose-stimulated insulin secretion. This has the effect of increasing hunger hormones called *ghrelin* and subsequently causing obesity. Other research[37] shows that production of another metabolite (called *succinate*) by bacteria can help in improving glucose metabolism and that bacterial fermentation of dietary fiber produces large amounts of succinate. This could mean that eating more fiber in a way that will promote more production of succinate by bacteria could improve glucose metabolism and in turn help to reverse or prevent metabolic syndrome.

Interestingly, when a fecal microbiome sample from lean, healthy people was transplanted into individuals suffering from glucose intolerance, the recipients gradually improved their insulin sensitivity. The effects were only temporary, disappearing after a few weeks, but this demonstrated that gut bacteria influences the conditions that cause metabolic syndrome and may be one of the solutions.[38]

- **Response to red meat.** An interesting study showed that the harmful cardiovascular effects of eating red meat could be due to the way the microbiome responds to it.[39] This research suggests that when people eat red meat, they don't all process it the same way, in part because of individual microbiome variations. Red meat contains L-carnitine, which can be processed, by a series of steps in the microbiome and then in the host, into a substance called *trimethylamine N-oxide* (TMAO); this substance alters the metabolism of cholesterol and slows the removal of cholesterol from the blood, contributing to its accumulation on artery walls.

  The interesting finding is that the conversion of L-carnitine to TMAO requires an intermediate substance and processing step that is accomplished only by gut bacteria. People who do not have the proper gut bacteria to convert L-carnitine into TMAO are at lower risk for cholesterol accumulation in the arteries. Vegetarians typically have less of these bacteria, so they do not get the TMAO conversion that meat eaters get after consuming red meat. This, of course, was big news in the media because it provided ammunition for following a vegetarian diet, although vegetarians typically would not eat red meat anyway.[40,41] This is another example of how individuals react differently to different foods—red meat is more harmful to some than to others. In this case, the personalization element seems to be determined specifically by the microbiome.

Consumption of red meat can cause heart disease in a way that is mediated by and depends on the microbiome.

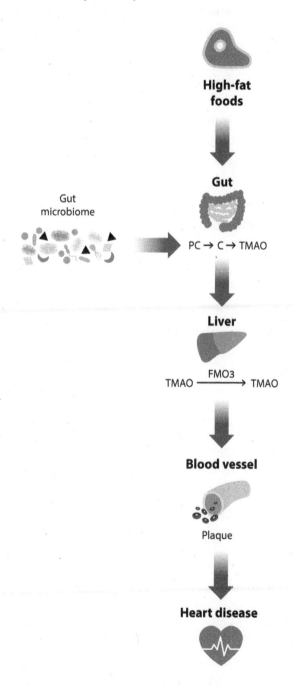

Your Unique Microbiome Signature

There are some bacteria in the microbiome that most humans have in common (considered the "core" of our microbiome), and there are some that may be inherited,[42] but there are also many that are only in their particular configuration inside you, creating a sort of microbiome "signature" that is all your own. Yours may be more similar to your relatives than to strangers, but it is still unique to you. For example, the microbiomes of identical twins are somewhat more similar than those of fraternal twins, which in turn are more similar than those in siblings, which are more similar than those in unrelated individuals, but identical twin microbiomes are still distinct from one another. Your microbiome is your personal and dynamic signature, constantly evolving and changing in response to your environment, and changes according to what you eat, your health status, and how you live. But it always retains certain personal elements that change very slowly in response to dietary or other lifestyle adjustments.

Your Microbiome and Your Weight

If you are trying to lose weight, you may be eager to know if your microbiome can help—or if it is a source of the problem. We now know that there is a connection between weight and the microbiome, but we are still studying many of the details about how that connection works. Much of what we know is because of research with obese mice. Specifically, we know that the microbiomes of obese mice are distinct from the microbiomes of normal-weight mice in several ways.

Obese mice extract more calories out of the same food, compared to non-obese mice. When the feces from obese mice was transferred into "germ-free mice" (sterile mice with no microbiome), essentially transplanting these mice with the microbiome of obese mice, those mice became obese.[43] This suggests that the microbiome has a strong effect on whether someone tends to be overweight.

This effect was also observed when microbiome samples from obese humans were transferred to germ-free mice. The microbiomes from sets of identical twin females, one obese and one lean, were transplanted into mice, and the germ-free mouse receiving the microbiome from the obese twin became obese (see the following figure). The mouse receiving the microbiome from the lean twin did not become obese.[44] Another interesting finding from this study was that co-housing the mice (those that received the microbiome of the obese female twin and those that received the microbiome of the lean female twin) did not result in obesity, although mice in captivity typically transfer their microbiomes from one to another by consuming each other's feces. In this case, because all the mice had microbiomes in place (as opposed to transplanting a microbiome into a mouse without one), the microbiomes of the various mice competed with the ingested feces and could overcome any obesity effects. This is evidence that some components in the microbiome might also protect from obesity.

This research suggests that the microbiome is at least a contributing factor to obesity, and probably in many ways. But what is even more interesting is how the microbiome affects what we try to *do* about our weight.

Transplanting the microbiome of identical twins discordant for obesity into mice transfers the obesity phenotype.

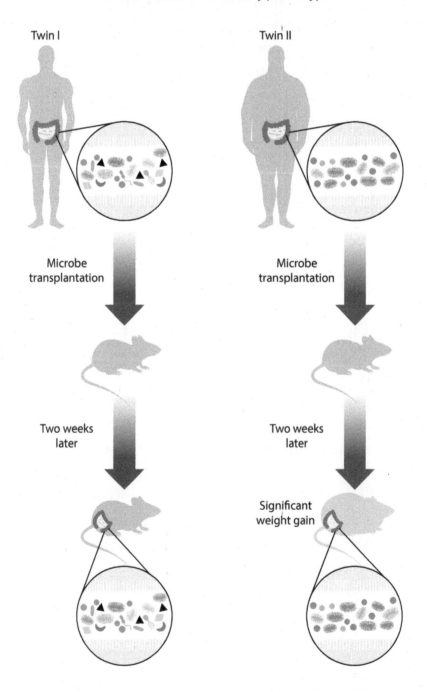

How Scientists Research the Microbiome

Scientists study the microbiome in a variety of ways. One is by studying mice. Mice have an advantage in that they can be used for establishing causality—in other words, they make it easy to determine that one thing causes another thing. Special germ-free mice that have had their microbiomes completely wiped out are like a clean slate. These mice can be implanted with specific microbes, to see what happens. Scientists can observe changes in the phenotype (the things you can actually observe or measure in an organism, such as weight, glucose tolerance, insulin resistance, blood chemistry, etc.), and this can help prove what the microbiome does and does not influence.

The other way scientists study the microbiome is through observational studies in humans. This more accurately establishes correlation—for example, whether a microbiome configuration correlates with a certain observable trait, like obesity or diabetes. This observation doesn't mean that a particular microbiome configuration *causes* obesity. It just shows the two patterns exist together. There are ways to assess causality. A study can look at the same person a variety of times (this is called adding a longitudinal dimension). This may help to establish which came first: a change in the microbiome or a change in the phenotype (like obesity or diabetes). Although this type of study doesn't definitively prove causality, it gets close enough to allow us to form hypotheses, which we can go on to test through additional research.

Research Spotlight: Microbiome Effects on Yo-Yo Dieting and Weight Regain[45]

One of the many questions that intrigues us about weight battles for people is, why do so many dieters who lose weight eventually experience weight rebound? They may lose anywhere between 5 and 50 or more pounds, but more often than not, they gain most of it back. Worse still, the clear majority of recurrently obese individuals not only return to their pre-dieting overweight but also regain more weight with each dieting cycle. During each such dieting–weight regain cycle, their proportion of body fat increases, and so does their risk of developing metabolic disorders, including adult-onset diabetes, fatty liver, and other obesity-related diseases.

Anyone who has dieted knows about this weight-regain phenomenon, either through experience or because they have seen it happen to others and worry it is going to happen to them. And in most cases, it does. While there are many different statistics available about how many diets fail, our research revealed to us that approximately 80 percent of people who lost weight regained it, and sometimes gained more than they lost. Those aren't good odds for hopeful dieters. This phenomenon is sometimes called *recurrent obesity*, or more often, *yo-yo dieting* or *yo-yo obesity*.

There are few things more frustrating to someone trying to get control of their weight and health than a seeming inability to keep off the weight that was so difficult to lose. We wanted to know why this happens. Our hypothesis was that if people experience a weight rebound, then somehow their bodies must "remember" the previous state of being overweight, creating an environment in which their bodies tended to want to revert to that previous state. But where would such a tendency or memory be stored? Gene activity could be responsible somehow. Or it's possible that different immunological or physiological alterations that happened when someone became obese don't fully return to what they were before obesity, after weight loss. This could make it more difficult for a body to retain the postobese, newly lean state.

We also thought that perhaps this "memory" might be stored in the microbiome. After all, we know the microbiome responds constantly to our diets and other changing conditions. We also know, from our own previous work and from the work of others, that during a state of obesity and weight gain, the microbiome changes distinctly. We also know this later state can lead to metabolic disruptions. For example, as we've already discussed, the microbiome begins extracting more energy (calories) from the same food in a state of obesity.

So, what if the microbiome, which was altered during the obese state, did *not* return, or return fully, to its previous lean-body configuration after weight loss? What if the body was lean but the microbiome maintained its obese configuration and was therefore making weight maintenance more difficult? And what would this look like, in terms of the actual bacterial species in the microbiome? Nobody had ever suggested this before, but it was an idea we were willing to put effort and resources into studying. And sure enough, our efforts paid off.

This line of thinking was the impetus for our mouse study on yo-yo obesity. The first thing we did was to take a group of mice and put them on a weight-gain diet to make them obese. Then we forced them to lose weight until their diets were successful (i.e., their weights returned to the same levels as those of mice of the same age and gender that had never become obese). Next we gave both groups of mice—that now had identical ages and weights—the same weight-gain diet. We were basically encouraging weight regain in the mice that had lost weight and encouraging weight gain in the mice that had never been obese. Interestingly, the group of mice that had a history of obesity and enforced weight loss gained more weight than the control group of mice that had never been obese, although they were eating an identical diet. In other words, the previously obese mice *regained more weight* from a diet that did not cause excessive weight gain in the other group.

When we subjected this "yo-yo dieting" group to another cycle of weight loss, followed by a third round of a weight-gain diet, the weight gain in the formerly obese mice was even more exacerbated, so that each series of weight regain seemed to induce more weight gain than the previous one. This mimicked yo-yo dieting in people, when they go on successive diets, losing and then regaining weight.

To confirm exactly where and how the yo-yo mice had encoded a "memory" of being obese, we first compared the two groups of mice (the ones that successfully dieted back to normal weight and the ones that were never obese to start with) across many clinical parameters: glucose metabolism, body fat, insulin sensitivity, liver function, and many other measures. We found no significant difference between the two groups of mice, in any of these areas... except in their microbiomes.

At the primary phase of the experiment, when the mice first gained weight, their microbiomes indeed became different from that of the lean mice. But when the mice dieted and returned to normal weight levels, their "obese" microbiomes remained altered in the obese state. This supported our theory that the obesity "memory" was stored in the microbiome. Because the microbiomes of obese mice and humans extract more calories from food than the microbiomes of lean mice and humans, we believe this is the reason the microbiomes of the yo-yo mice "remembered" being obese by retaining their tendency to extract more calories from food (see the following figure).

Additionally, when we continued to feed the previously obese mice a normal diet, it took many months—the potential equivalent of *years* in humans—for their bodies and their microbiomes to equilibrate back to the lean state. Once the microbiomes did equilibrate, a second round of the fattening diet did not cause

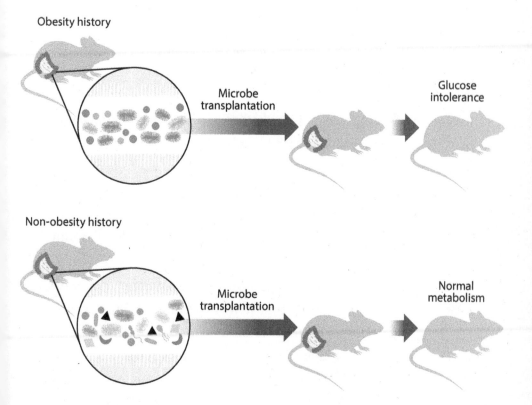

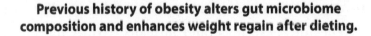

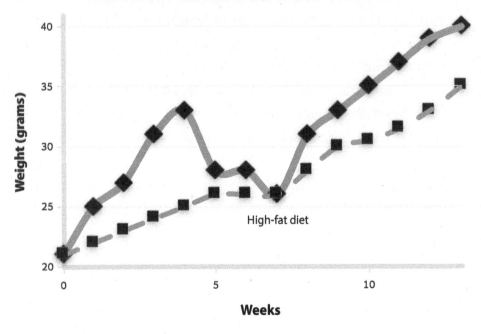

Previous history of obesity alters gut microbiome composition and enhances weight regain after dieting.

exacerbated weight gain. They had regained a microbiome state of a truly lean mouse—but it took a long time.

If you were to extrapolate this study to humans, you could say that once you have been overweight, it will take you months to years to get your microbiome back to the state of a lean person. Until that happens, you may not be able to eat the same amount of food as an always-lean person and maintain your weight loss.

But so far, we had discovered only an association, not causation. We didn't yet prove that it was the microbiome causing the weight gain. We had to develop a way to determine that it was indeed the microbiome of the mice, not something else that was causing this effect. We needed to wipe out or reboot their microbiomes and did this by treating the mice with antibiotics.

Just as we had hoped, the antibiotic treatment completely abolished the effect of being formerly obese! After the antibiotic treatment, the mice with a previous history of obesity no longer gained more weight than the controls.

We wanted to be thorough, so next we moved to testing our theories with germ-free mice. These are specialized mice used in research that have no microbiomes. They are housed in sterile isolators, ensuring that they do not take on any intestinal bacteria before the experiment. We transplanted fecal samples from the previously obese mice into the germ-free mice without microbiomes, and sure enough, after the transfer, these formerly microbiome-free mice experienced accelerated weight regain, as if they had formerly been obese. This was a final confirmation for our theory—at least in mice—that the microbiome was the cause of the postdieting accelerated weight gain and yo-yo obesity.

At the conclusion of this study, we were able to develop a machine-learning algorithm, based on hundreds of personalized microbiome parameters (such as which microbes the microbiome contained and what those microbes do), which could accurately predict exactly how much weight each mouse (whether formerly obese or always lean) would gain on the high-calorie, fattening diet.

If the story (and the research) ended there, it would be a little discouraging. This was not a human study, and remember our previous cautions to oversimplify the conclusions of research? But you may be tempted to conclude that like the mice, once you have been obese, you will never be able to eat normally again, or at best, you will have to diet stringently for years. But what if this obesity effect could be modified in some easy way? That was our next question, so we began to investigate the differences in the microbiomes between lean and obese mice. Could there be something we could use?

One thing we noticed was that the yo-yo mice had significantly lower flavonoid levels (specifically the molecules apigenin and naringenin) than the mice that had always been lean. One of the things flavonoids do is help your fat cells burn more calories. We theorized that the low levels of these flavonoids during weight cycling might contribute to the formerly obese mice's tendency to extract more calories from food than lean mice.

We wondered what would happen if we provided a dietary source of flavonoids to the yo-yo mice. Flavonoids are the chemicals typically found in vegetables as well as in berries, tree fruits, nuts and beans, and spices, so they are widely available in the food supply as well as in supplement form. We were very excited to see that this postbiotic treatment *cured the mice of enhanced weight regain.*

"Postbiotics"

We coined the term *postbiotics* to describe metabolites that are, or should be, produced by bacteria in the microbiome and that can in turn affect human cells and can be administered in supplement form. Just as prebiotic supplements containing beneficial bacteria and prebiotic fiber can be administered as supplements, postbiotics can target specific microbiome deficiencies. We were able to demonstrate that by intervening at this postbiotic level—that is, by supplying the host with molecules that are produced by bacteria—we could affect cell processes and biological conditions, such as excessive weight regain. This allows us to intervene in the microbiome/host interaction at a completely new level.

Before you run out and spend your money on flavonoid supplements, we must say that this benefit has not yet been shown in humans. Although mouse studies can be suggestive, they do not prove that humans will react the same way. However, it certainly couldn't hurt to eat more flavonoid-rich vegetables during and after dieting—specifically those containing higher levels of apigenin and naringenin. Sources of apigenin include chamomile tea, onions, oranges, grapefruit, celery, parsley, and cilantro, as well as red wine and beer, while sources of naringenin include citrus and citrus juice, almonds, pistachios, and again, red wine. There isn't really a downside to eating these nutrient-dense foods.

We are now conducting similar studies in people. We hope to discover the specific compounds that may help revert this bad microbial "memory" in the human gut and help maintain normal weight after successfully dieting. Keep an eye out for this future information, which should be even more useful in developing effective microbiome-altering therapies.

Microbiome Messaging

Your microbiome does not exist in isolation inside your gut. In fact, it "talks" to the rest of your body in some intriguing ways we are only beginning to understand. Some findings out of our own research labs showed that the gut microbiome communicates with other parts of the body, like fat tissue, the liver, pancreas, cardiovascular system, lungs, and the brain. This could potentially influence a huge range of health issues, like the tendency toward or protection against obesity, insulin resistance, liver disease, diabetes, heart disease, allergies, asthma, and even behavioral problems, by influencing how the cells in the body behave. This can affect the way the cells and also the genes behave.

Microbiome Influences

We've already seen how dieting and overeating can potentially affect the microbiome, but so can being exposed to another person or animal or a new environment. This could be kissing someone, petting a dog or cat, or taking a swim in the ocean; the composition of your microbiome is affected. Although your microbiome signature is unique, it also changes constantly—not all of it, but enough to make a difference in how your microbiome functions and affects your health and life. Some of the influences on your microbiome are inherited or happened long ago, and some are current, such as the following:

Significant Influences

- **Evolution:** Animals whose diets diverged from those of their ancestors have microbiomes that have adapted to the new diets.[46,47,48,49]
- **Age:** We are all born sterile (without microbiomes) and pick up our first microbes from our parents, starting during our trek through the birth canal and our first feeding, and then from our immediate environments. Infants have very different microbiomes than adults. When they begin to eat solid food, their microbiomes slowly change to become more like those of adults in general.[50,51,52] This process usually ends at the age of three, when the microbiome of a child roughly resembles that of an adult.
- **Traditional versus modern lifestyle:** People who live traditional lifestyles, like hunter-gatherers or farmers who use traditional agricultural techniques, have much more microbiome diversity than people living a more modern

life.[53,54] (Diversity in the microbiome is good and usually results in more vigorous health.)

Moderate Influences

- **Antibiotic use:** Antibiotics are one of the greatest medical discoveries of the twentieth century. They have dramatically contributed to human health and longevity, because they are an effective treatment for what was once the greatest human killer: infectious disease. This triumph also comes at a price—antibiotics have a long-term effect on the microbiome, including reducing diversity, although individuals respond differently to antibiotic use.[55,56,57,58] As such, antibiotic treatment that is not medically indicated (such as when you use antibiotics to treat a cold or any other situation when they aren't needed), as well as antibiotics in food from inoculating livestock, may induce harm by altering our healthy microbiome.
- **Fiber intake:** Those who consume more fiber tend to have more microbiome diversity than those who consume a low-fiber diet, although this diversity can be at least partially recovered by changing to a high-fiber diet.[59,60]
- **Exposure to drugs (other than antibiotics):** Drugs many people take regularly, such as acetaminophen, proton-pump inhibitors, and metformin, alter the microbiome, and that alteration may contribute to the side effects you experience from a drug.[61,62,63,64,65] In fact, it was recently suggested that the variable response of people to the same drugs may be caused by their different microbiomes. This may even hold true for anticancer drugs that prove useful to some patients but not to others. (Personalized medicine

is another vibrant area of research right now, including personalized cancer treatment.[66])

- **Genetics:** As we mentioned earlier, while identical twins do not have identical microbiomes, their microbiomes are somewhat more similar than those of fraternal twins. Some groups of bacteria may be heritable, and even those microbes that have evolved within an ancestral group may remain and continue to benefit you more than microbes you acquired only recently, such as within your own lifetime.[67,68,69] However, the extent by which our genetic makeup determines how our microbiome looks remains unknown and is the subject of intense scientific research (including our own).

- **Exercise:** Extreme athletes have different microbiomes than others who are the same sex, age, and weight. Some of this variation may be due to their consuming different diets, but studies involving mice suggest that exercise alone has an impact on microbiome composition.[70,71,72]

- **Roommates and pets:** People who live together share microbiome features, and pets also affect microbiomes, although pet effects tend to be most concentrated on skin microbes rather than gut microbes.[73]

Minor but Still Significant Influences

- **Short-term dietary changes:** What you eat today, or when you are on a short-term diet, or when traveling, or other temporary changes to your diet have an effect on your microbiome, but if you resume your regular way of eating, your microbiome also tends to revert.[74,75] This is similar to what we saw in our bread study: short-term changes to the microbiome matched the long-term changes of long-term bread eaters.

Fecal Transplants: Cutting-Edge Science or a Dangerous Experiment?

Can you imagine transplanting someone else's feces into your lower intestine? Believe it or not, this is new and innovative science and has already been an effective treatment for some people with certain serious intestinal conditions like recurrent *C. diff*. The treatment is just like it sounds: Feces from a healthy person is implanted into the rectum of an unhealthy person, and the theory is that this lends good bacteria from the donor that can help edge out the bad guys that are causing problems in the person who is sick. There are also other means of taking the fecal microbiota transplantation (FMT), such as in pill form, although traditionally, the transplant goes directly into the colon.

When this treatment has been used to treat patients suffering from antibiotic-resistant *C. diff*, more than 90 percent of cases resolved within weeks—which is astonishing! It also has been used to resolve some cases of ulcerative colitis. This is significant because *C. diff* is a worldwide problem, and while antibiotics are the first line of treatment, many cases are antibiotic-resistant and recurring. In these instances, FMTs have become the next wave in the fight. It really seems to work like magic (although currently only for resolving *C. diff* infections)—someone suffering for months with this condition and at a serious risk of dying is completely cured by the treatment.

A similar approach has been attempted in resolving some other diseases, such as ulcerative colitis, diabetes, Crohn's disease, inflammatory bowel disease (IBD), and even metabolic syndrome, mentioned earlier, but the results of these experiments involving chronic disorders have been more variable. It has even been suggested that the response to FMT is personalized! Some people react better to transplants from some donors than to others. This suggests (and we will discuss this in more detail in the following sections) that the microbiome is a strong determinant affecting our individualized response to food and to medical treatment.

Fecal transfer is a highly regulated process; doctors must get permission to use the treatment, and so far, it is only approved to treat C. diff, but it is an expanding area of research. A company called OpenBiome, which collects and stores donated stool samples from healthy people, has provided more than 16,000 treatments to clinicians at more than 700 medical centers in every U.S. state and in six countries. However, it is far from standard treatment, and there is currently no indication that FMT will be successful, or reliably successful, for any condition other than C. diff. Still, many are hopeful that this treatment could be expanded. It is an active area of research.

In the meantime, don't try this at home! FMT is a rather aggressive, crude, and somewhat uncontrolled method of modulating the microbiome. There are stories about people doing this on their own, but you can't be sure exactly what the donor fecal sample contains, and you might transmit pathogenic bacteria to yourself, or theoretically, you could even transmit the donor's tendency to develop disease. One such example is a woman who was successfully treated for a C. diff infection with a fecal transplant from her obese daughter. The woman rapidly gained 30 pounds after the procedure, becoming obese herself. Whether this was a direct complication of her FMT remains to be seen. Unfortunately, any positive results from transferring fecal samples from lean donors to obese donors seems to be very temporary, at least in studies published so far.

The idea that FMTs may someday wipe out intestinal infections and cure obesity is exciting and promising, but we aren't there yet. To really understand and control what we are doing when we use FMT, we need a better mechanistic understanding of how it works, and more research and practice. With such knowledge, we may be able to envision a future in which microbes or their products will be transplanted, rather than transplanting a person's entire gut microbiome.

Research Spotlight: Circadian Rhythms[76]

Circadian-rhythm disruption is one of the results of modern technology and can cause some problems for health. We have already seen evidence that night-shift workers have an increased risk of obesity,[77] heart attack,[78] and breast cancer.[79] One 2011 study even showed that if you work the night shift for ten years or more, you boost your risk for type 2 diabetes by 40 percent.[80] But the link between shift work and disease remained unclear for many decades. Because there are tens of millions of shift workers in multiple professions (22.5 million or more in Europe and more than 15 million in the United States) as well as frequent flyers across time zones and millions of people experiencing chronic sleep disturbances that are likely affected by circadian-rhythm disruption, we felt this was an important issue to understand better, and it also intrigued us.

Being heavily involved in microbiome research, we thought that it could certainly be possible that the microbiome would not be immune to the dramatic changes in gene activity that accompany circadian activity. Because circadian rhythms are linked to light exposure, and your microbes hang out in the dark of your gut, you might not think the microbiome could have much to do with circadian rhythms. However, we wondered if maybe, because bacteria thrive directly on the food available to them, and food intake typically changes between day and night, there might be a circadian rhythm and microbiome connection. Typically, we eat in the day and sleep at night. Our digestive processes are different during these time periods, so these differences might also have a profound effect on the microbiome. We thought it sounded plausible, and we decided to study it. We didn't know if we would find anything at all, but this is part of the thrill of research—to study and experiment with what no one has ever experimented with before. We hit quite a gold mine.

Surprisingly, we found that the human microbiome follows its own circadian rhythm, and its rhythm is controlled both by our own internal human biological clock and by our eating schedule and patterns. Those bacteria are aware of this rhythm and respond in concert with your response. Specifically, we found that some microbes are more abundant in the morning, meaning they are growing and replicating more, and others are more abundant at night, when they grow and replicate more. If an organism changes its sleep/wake cycle—and therefore its cycle of eating—would the microbiome alter in response?

To find out, we conducted an experiment using mice. We began by essentially making them "work the graveyard shift" by keeping them awake when they would normally sleep, essentially "jet lagging" them by 8 hours. Mice are nocturnal, so in this case, we had to keep them awake during the day and let them sleep only at night.

In the presence of this artificially induced jet lag, we recorded notable changes in the mouse microbiomes, such that the mice were thrown into a state of dysbiosis, meaning their microbiota stopped functioning correctly, causing measurable health changes. We saw changes in both microbiome composition and function; consequently, the mice became far less efficient at cell growth, DNA repair, and detoxification, and developed both obesity and glucose intolerance[81]—the same way shift workers do. We were also able to transfer the jet-lagged bacteria into germ-free mice, and they, too, became obese and developed glucose intolerance.

This theory is much harder to test in humans, of course, but we did study a small number of people while they were traveling all over the world, including to and from the United States and the Far East. This travel induced an approximately 8-hour jet lag similar to what we induced in the mice. (We were very popular on campus, offering students a free round-trip plane ticket to the United States in exchange for a few fecal samples.) We sampled the gut bacteria of these people three times over two weeks, capturing the main stages of jet lag, and we found that their microbes changed in composition and in ways that were startlingly similar. Additionally, we transferred the humans' jet-lagged bugs into germ-free mice, and we could clearly see that transferring the gut microbes from the point where jet lag was at its highest induced much more obesity and glucose intolerance.

We were relieved to find that the gut microbes of the travelers returned to normal two weeks after their flights, and transferring their bugs into mice at that time no longer led to increased obesity and glucose intolerance. In our view, our work finally provides at least a partial explanation for the epidemiological observation that shift workers are more prone to the metabolic syndrome. Interestingly, in follow-up studies, we discovered that the microbiome circadian rhythm is tightly linked to that of the host. In fact, we've recently shown that by altering the microbiome rhythm in mice, we can affect the diurnal function of organs, such as the liver, thereby affecting their capacity to break down chemicals and medications.[82]

While the impact of circadian-rhythm disruption is clear, making changes like turning down a lucrative night-shift job, refusing a transcontinental trip, or going to bed at sunset and getting up at sunrise are not practical options and wouldn't allow you to take advantage of many of the modern pleasures of life. However, our point is that the more we learn about how the microbiome is influenced by circadian rhythms, the better we will be able to understand how we might modify these effects through other means than reverting to strictly rising and setting with the sun.

Research Spotlight: Artificial Sweeteners[83]

We've already talked briefly about the link between artificial sweeteners and weight gain, but in case you are still consuming diet soda, or if you want to know more, we have done specific research into the effect artificial sweeteners can have on the microbiome.

As with shift work, there has been prior suggestion that consuming noncaloric artificial sweeteners (NAS) is associated with obesity and diabetes. This is counterintuitive because these sweeteners have no calories, and there have been many claims, by dieters as well as national organizations, that artificial sweeteners can assist with weight loss by reducing calorie intake. We wanted to find out why so many research studies support the idea that a zero-calorie product would contribute to weight gain and associated blood sugar disturbances. We all know that many people who are overweight drink diet soda, but most people probably assume this is an attempt at losing weight, not the cause of the excess weight.

Before we started our research, we did a little background investigation. As we've already mentioned, the official position statement of the American Heart Association and the American Diabetes Association on non-nutritive sweeteners supports their use, stating the following in 2012:[84]

- Substituting non-nutritive sweeteners for sugars added to foods and beverages may help people reach and maintain a healthy body weight—as long as the substitution doesn't lead to eating additional calories later as "compensation."
- For people with diabetes, non-nutritive sweeteners used alone or in foods and beverages remain an option and when used appropriately can aid in glucose control.
- Substituting non-nutritive sweeteners for added sugars in beverages and other foods has the potential to help people reach and maintain a healthy body weight and help people with diabetes with glucose control.

The rationale behind this declaration is seemingly understandable. The sweetening power of most low-calorie artificial sweeteners is at least 100 times more intense than regular sugar, so only a small amount is needed when you use these sugar substitutes. Thus, with a smaller amount one can satisfy the sweet tooth craving, and do so with fewer calories. So shouldn't fewer calories translate to less weight gain, or more weight loss?

Moreover, with the exception of aspartame, noncaloric artificial sweeteners cannot be broken down by the body. This is what makes them "noncaloric." Our bodies cannot extract energy from them. They give us the sweet taste we crave and then pass through our systems without being digested, so how could they have much effect?

And yet, this very argument was the crux of our hypothesis, prompting our research on artificial sweeteners and the microbiome: Food and nutrients like fiber (and certain chemicals, like artificial sweeteners) that pass out of the stomach undigested pass *into the microbiome* undigested, meaning they are more likely to influence the action of the microbiome in a way for which the microbiome may be unprepared. The microbiome is used to receiving undigested fiber, which it consumes as food (fiber is a prebiotic). But what would it do with artificial sweeteners? We suspected that artificial sweeteners could potentially be toxic to the bacteria, and might even kill beneficial species. Or, maybe some gut microbes digest some of the artificial sweetener, producing unfamiliar metabolites that could be taken up by the person and influence health in some way. Whatever the mechanism, nobody had ever asked the question before, so we decided to ask and try to find the answer.

We added high doses (but not higher than the amounts currently allowed by the FDA, when calibrated from human weight to mouse weight) of the three most commonly used artificial sweeteners—aspartame, sucralose, and saccharin—to the drinking water of mice. After several weeks of drinking water supplemented with these artificial sweeteners, we were startled to see a dramatic effect: Most of the mice became glucose intolerant, which means that their ability to metabolize glucose was greatly reduced. (Glucose intolerance is the hallmark of diabetes.)

We were surprised that no one had seen the potential link between artificial sweeteners and glucose intolerance. Being skeptical scientists, at first we did not believe what we saw, so we asked our students to repeat the experiments. We saw the same results. It seemed that one of the easiest and most direct ways to induce glucose intolerance in mice was to feed them artificial sweeteners!

At this point, it was clear that something interesting was going on because in this controlled environment, artificial sweeteners were obviously having adverse metabolic effects.

Consumption of noncaloric artificial sweeteners alters the composition and function of the microbiome and can induce glucose intolerance in the mouse or human host.

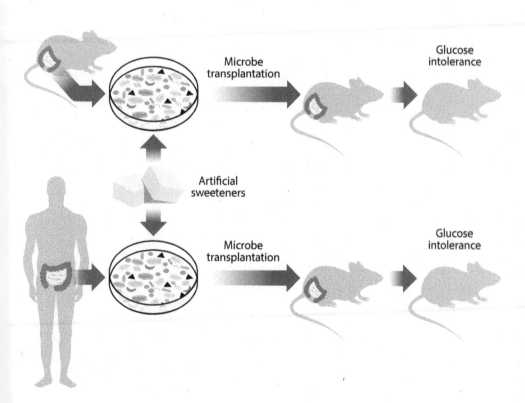

We wanted to study this surprising phenomenon better and focused on one of the three commonly used sweeteners, saccharin. We repeated the experiments with saccharin, using a group of mice with different genetic backgrounds and with different diets, and had the same results. We gradually reduced the levels of saccharin given to mice, but even at low levels, the mice still developed glucose intolerance. The lowest doses of saccharin inducing these adverse effects were comparable to normal consumption of a person using artificial sweeteners in diet sodas or coffee.

We still didn't understand why artificial sweeteners were having this effect, so we decided to experiment further. Next, we tested the hypothesis that the gut microbiota is involved in this phenomenon. We thought the bacteria might cause this glucose intolerance as a reaction to artificial sweeteners, which the body may not recognize as food. To do this, we first treated mice with antibiotics to eradicate their microbiomes—and this resulted in a *full reversal of the artificial sweeteners' effects on glucose metabolism!* This was a first and quite compelling sign that the microbiome was indeed involved in glucose metabolism, but we didn't stop there.

Next, we transferred the microbiota from mice that consumed artificial sweeteners to "germ free" mice, and this resulted in a complete transmission of the glucose intolerance into the recipient mice. This was conclusive proof that changes to the gut bacteria are involved in the harmful effects of artificial sweeteners.

Finally, we did the ultimate experiment—we took the microbiota of normal mice who had never consumed artificial sweeteners, and we grew it in vials, kept outside the body, in the presence of artificial sweeteners, to eliminate the influence of any other elements. We then transferred this externally grown microbiota into germ-free mice. We wondered what might happen to mice that had never consumed artificial sweeteners, if they were exposed to bacteria that had consumed artificial sweeteners. This, too, induced glucose intolerance in the germ-free mice. We were increasingly convinced of the major negative impact of artificial sweeteners on gut bacteria!

A detailed characterization of the microbiota in these mice revealed profound changes to their bacterial populations, including developing microbial functions that are known to cause a propensity for obesity, diabetes, and complications of these problems in both mice and humans.

We were still not fully satisfied, maybe because the results still seemed so surprising. We wanted to know if the effect would translate to humans, so we conducted a small-scale controlled experiment. We asked a group of volunteers who did not normally eat or drink artificially sweetened foods to consume them for a week. We took microbiome samples and tested fasting blood sugar levels for each participant at the beginning of the study. Then they all logged everything they ate, including the artificial sweeteners, on a mobile app we developed. After the week was over, we retested everyone's microbiome and blood sugar level. The findings showed that about half of the volunteers had begun to develop glucose intolerance after *only one week* of artificial sweetener consumption at levels currently allowed by the FDA! We find this startling and cause for more aggressive investigation into the safety of this additive. Also, notice that half responded dramatically to the artificial sweeteners—but half did not.

The composition of their gut microbiota explained the difference: We discovered two different populations of human gut bacteria—one that induced glucose intolerance when exposed to the artificial sweeteners and a second that seemed to disregard the artificial sweeteners completely. We also discovered that we could predict, based on the microbiome samples we took prior to artificial sweetener consumption, which individuals would respond negatively to the artificial sweetener, before they ever consumed any.

Based on our research, we believe that certain bacteria in the guts of those who developed glucose intolerance reacted to the chemical sweeteners by secreting metabolites that then provoked an inflammatory response like what would happen in some people after eating a large amount of sugar. This promoted measurable changes in the body's ability to utilize sugar. Although the artificial sweetener was not sugar and did not contain calories, its microbiome effect was still quite similar, as if the microbiome perceived the artificial sweeteners as sugar, regardless of calorie content.

This research got quite a lot of international publicity. The results were quite conclusive that we believe they justify conducting large-scale human trials as part of a reassessment of official recommendations about artificial sweeteners, whose results may merit reassessment of today's massive, unregulated consumption of artificially sweetened products.

As for us personally, we both used artificial sweeteners in our coffee and drank diet soda, and never thought they were harmful. We thought they were beneficial. But given our surprising results, we have decided not to use them anymore, and we know many other people who have also stopped using them after reading our study. (Note for the curious: Stevia is not an artificial sweetener, and we did not study stevia.)

We also believe that because there were a few people whose gut bacteria did not react to the sweeteners, this research is also further proof of the necessity of nutritional personalization, especially taking into consideration each person's unique microbiome configuration. Companies that can profile people's microbiomes are now emerging and performing this test affordably, so soon you may be able to find out for yourself if you tolerate these sweeteners or not. Until then, however, we believe that playing the odds will pay off for most people. Better to stop drinking diet soda, using artificial sweetener in coffee and tea, and eating foods with artificial sweeteners, until you know for sure that artificial sweeteners don't harm your metabolism. (But don't revert to sugar—it is equally harmful, in different ways! It would be much safer and healthier to drink water instead of soda.)

We still have much to learn about the microbiome, especially what we can do to manipulate it in our favor. We know fiber helps to cultivate a healthy microbiome, and we know that artificial sweeteners and certain lifestyles may have a negative impact. We have evidence that flavonoids may help to guard against weight regain, but we still don't know for sure whether probiotic supplements really do anything. Basically, we still have much to learn, so beyond eating fiber and avoiding artificial sweeteners, we still can't say anything for sure. We believe that by better understanding the role of the microbiome and the metabolites it produces in disease states, we will be able to design more targeted interventions that could specifically wipe out certain bacteria or introduce other bacteria that will help us. Perhaps someday, all this will be possible with capsules containing what our microbiomes need. But until then, we have another, more easily measured avenue for understanding personal responses, and microbiome responses, to the foods we eat and the way we live. That measure is blood sugar.

CHAPTER 6

Blood Sugar: Your Ultimate Food Feedback Response

Shay is an airline pilot with a regular flight schedule, and for years, he has followed the same daily routine. At the same time every day, he piloted a flight that went to the same place and then returned home that same day. The complete trip took several hours, so he always took a snack with him. He would eat the same snack (a sandwich) after the flight to the destination—but every time on the return flight, he always felt tired. This disturbed him, of course, because airline pilots must be alert and being fatigued made staying vigilant more difficult. He couldn't understand why he felt fatigued, because he was getting enough sleep and exercised regularly. He hoped he wasn't developing some sort of illness. Then he entered our study.

When Shay began tracking his blood sugar as part of our study, he discovered something surprising—every time he ate

175

bread, he experienced an extreme blood sugar spike. Bread does not have this effect on everyone. By now we also know (as we explained in Chapter 1) that even *different types* of bread may have different responses in different individuals. Some people eat bread, or a specific type of bread, and have only a mild blood sugar rise. Others get big spikes, and Shay was one of the latter, so it seemed a likely culprit for his afternoon fatigue. Shay decided to try switching his sandwich for a standard airplane meal, which usually contained starchy food, other than bread, like rice or pasta. After he made the switch in what he ate, his afternoon fatigue *completely disappeared*.

Could something as simple as exchanging bread for pasta or rice have such a dramatic effect on afternoon fatigue? A more precise question would be: Could something as simple as switching out bread for pasta or rice really have such a dramatic effect on blood sugar levels? The answer, of course, is *yes*.

Blood sugar is an important piece of the personal nutrition puzzle because it impacts your energy and fatigue levels (as was the case with Shay), but blood sugar instability (big highs, significant lows) can also negatively impact many aspects of your health. But what exactly is blood sugar, and why does it matter so much? Why do we keep talking about it, and why have we made it such a focus of our research? Here's what you need to know.

BLOOD SUGAR: YOUR PERSONAL FUEL SOURCE

Our bodies and brains run mostly on sugar, so you might think you need quite a lot. However, if your blood sugar is within normal range, you probably have only about five grams of sugar in your entire body—this translates to just over a teaspoon! But even such a small amount is crucial for your survival. A normal blood glucose level is 80 mg/dL. If your blood sugar fell below 60 mg/dL, you would have low blood sugar, or you would be in a hypoglycemic state. If your blood sugar dropped to 40 mg/dL (about half a teaspoon), you would likely start feeling dizzy and weak. A further drop could result in fainting, or possibly losing your life, if the situation was not quickly treated. On the other end of the spectrum, if you were diabetic and your blood sugar rose to dangerously high levels of 300 to 400 mg/dL (about 25 grams or 5 teaspoons), you would face health risks, both short-term and long-term.

To get an idea of how diet can influence sugar in your system, a 12-ounce can of non-diet soft drink of any kind contains 40 grams of sugar, or 8 teaspoons. That's enough to send your blood sugar well above the high diabetic range. A healthy body can manage an influx of a high amount of sugar like this on occasion, but multiple times daily may quickly tip the blood sugar balance into chronic unhealthy ranges, putting you at risk.

When you eat carbohydrates (whether from candy bars, bread, pasta, rice, fruit, or vegetables), your body converts carbs into glucose, which fuels your muscles, organs, and brain. Having blood sugar levels in a healthy range is crucial for functioning, and your body has intricate mechanisms to control blood sugar very tightly, in order to keep it within a narrow, beneficial range so you have enough for the energy you need—not too little (hypoglycemia), which could cause confusion, dizziness, shakiness, anxiety, seizures, and unconsciousness, and not too much (hyperglycemia), which could cause extreme thirst, excessive urination, weakness, confusion, dangerous pH blood imbalances, nerve damage, and even in some cases, diabetic coma and death.

Blood sugar control is a delicate balancing act that involves many systems in your body. Here's how the process works:

1. When you eat foods containing carbohydrates, your stomach acids and digestive enzymes break down and convert those sugars and starches into glucose.

2. When the glucose hits your small intestine, tiny hair-like projections called *microvilli* are amazingly efficient at absorbing the glucose and directing it into your bloodstream. How much goes into your blood depends on how much and what you ate. If you ate a large amount of any type of food, or if you ate certain types of carbohydrates, your blood sugar may go higher than normal—beyond the narrow range your body tries to maintain. This is called *postprandial* (or *postmeal*) *hyperglycemia*, or what we call a blood sugar spike.

3. As soon as your brain detects the presence of excess glucose in your blood, it sends a signal to your pancreas. Specialized cells termed *beta cells*, located in "islands" or tiny cell clusters within the pancreas (called *islets of Langerhans*), "feel" the body's sugar levels. They secrete insulin in small bursts throughout the day and release larger amounts of insulin following blood sugar surges after meals. These beta cells are crucial to sufficient insulin production and keeping blood sugar steady. In juvenile, insulin-dependent or type 1 diabetes, young people

develop intense inflammation in their islets of Langerhans that eventually leads to their destruction. To remain alive, people with type 1 diabetes need to inject insulin for the rest of their lives, as a replacement for their destroyed pancreatic beta cells. Insulin is like a key that unlocks the cells to receive glucose. If you eat a large amount of food, or consume certain carbohydrates, and your blood sugar level goes very high, your body may overreact by releasing too much insulin. This can make your blood sugar go too low (hypoglycemia). One of the symptoms of this is getting very hungry after eating, when you should be satiated. (In the next section, we will show you how to use hunger levels as one method for tracking blood sugar.)

4. While the pancreas controls insulin production, other organs, primarily the liver and muscles, use insulin to enable the consumption of blood sugar for energy. The liver, for example, takes up more glucose and converts it to glycogen, for storage. (Glycogen stores are quite limited. Even athletes can store only about 3,000 calories as glycogen.) Any remaining sugar that isn't used by the cells or the liver (and may be hanging around if your blood sugar went too high) or by other organs in the body (such as the muscles, heart, or brain) gets converted to fat and stored in fat cells. This is how blood sugar spikes can result in obesity—constant high blood sugar beyond what your body needs results in continual storage of that excess sugar as energy-rich fat in adipose cells. The more excess sugar you have in your blood, the bigger the fat stores you accumulate.

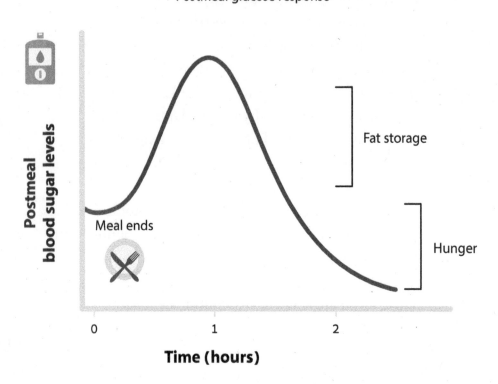

Postmeal glucose response

5. Once your blood sugar is stowed away, your body realizes that it needs more fuel (blood sugar), so you get hungry again. Normally, this should happen within about 3 or 4 hours of your last meal and just in time for your next feeding. When you eat something again, the cycle starts over.

When Blood Sugar Goes Too High

If you are healthy and you eat food that your system has evolved to manage, then your blood sugar control should work just fine. Only in rare cases does blood sugar control malfunction, such as with type 1 or juvenile diabetes. However, sometimes if people eat too much, or the wrong foods for too long, it can interfere with the body's blood sugar control system, causing blood sugar levels to get too high. In response, insulin can get too high, and this imbalance can cause a cascade of health problems.

Insulin Resistance

Chronically high blood sugar levels put stress on your whole system. This is especially true if you have a family tendency to have abnormal blood sugar control and/or type 2 diabetes. Eventually, this can result in a condition called *insulin resistance*, in which your body becomes desensitized to the effects of insulin. When you develop this condition, more insulin is required than before to get sugar out of your blood and into your cells. Because this destructive process often has no symptoms, insulin resistance has been called the "silent killer."[1] You may not know you have this condition until you have already suffered damage for many years, because you can't feel your glucose levels until they are extremely disrupted. At first, your pancreas reacts to your elevated blood sugar levels by increasing its insulin production. This excess insulin pushes most of the excess sugar into the cells and can partially normalize the high blood sugar levels. With time, this strenuous activity can cause the beta cells in your pancreas to become exhausted. Your pancreas reaches a point where it can no longer supply all the necessary insulin to maintain a decent blood sugar level, and this is when insulin resistance progresses to adult-onset, or type 2, diabetes.

An analogy we like to use is a thermostat and an air conditioner. An air conditioner with a thermostat is meant to keep your home at a fixed temperature, so when the temperature goes below a certain level, the air conditioner turns off, and when it goes above a certain level, the air conditioner turns on. However, if the front door is left open or the day is unusually hot, even a well-serviced air conditioner might have to run continuously and not be able to keep the room at a constant temperature, and eventually it may break down. In the same way, your body has mechanisms to keep blood sugar under control, but if your diet and lifestyle foil those mechanisms (you are "leaving the door open"), they can fail and create a destructive situation.

Insulin-Producing Beta Cell Death

While we still aren't completely sure about what kills beta cells in chronic adult-onset diabetes, high blood sugar probably greatly contributes to this deterioration:

- One study showed that in people whose blood sugar rose only slightly over 100 mg/dL 2 hours after a glucose tolerance test, there was already detectable beta cell dysfunction, and with every small increase in blood sugar at the 2-hour mark, the beta cell failure became more evident.[2]
- Another study showed that in people with only slightly higher-than-normal blood sugar (with fasting blood sugar between 110 and 125 mg/dL), there was a loss of an average of 40 percent of their beta cells.[3]
- Yet another study showed that when mice received beta cell transplants, those cells survived much better when the mouse's blood sugar stayed under 150 mg/dL. In those whose blood sugar rose above 150 mg/dL, there was a much higher level of transplanted beta cell death.

Metabolic Syndrome

In many cases, people suffering from insulin resistance also develop several co-occurring conditions, including obesity (especially around the waistline), high blood pressure, high triglycerides, high cholesterol, and accumulation of fat in the liver cells (termed *fatty liver*). Collectively, this defines a condition called *metabolic syndrome*. Close to 40 percent of the adult population in the United States suffers from one or more features of the metabolic syndrome. Although there are no physical symptoms that you can "feel," it is a dangerous condition that predisposes you to many different serious health issues, from diabetes to heart disease. As we've discussed in Chapter 2, the metabolic syndrome epidemic affecting our species in the last century has been closely linked with many nutritional and lifestyle changes that we took on ourselves with modernization, and many of these changes have drastically impacted our gut microbiome, with a ripple effect throughout the entire body.

Prediabetes

If it takes longer than normal for your body to get blood sugar under control and requires extra insulin to make that happen, you may be prediabetic. Officially, the diagnosis occurs when fasting blood sugar levels are regularly between 100 and 125 mg/dL. It is a serious condition because people with prediabetes are likely to progress to type 2 diabetes within a few years. This is also a common and often undiagnosed condition—an estimated 470 million people in the Western world will have prediabetes by the year 2030,[4] and many of them may never know until they have advanced to full-blown diabetes. Being prediabetic is also something you can't feel. You may not have any noticeable symptoms, which is why people tend to go undiagnosed for many years.

Type 2 Diabetes

Once blood sugar reaches a certain level—for example, two or more tests showing fasting blood sugar levels of 126 mg/dL or higher—type 2 diabetes is the diagnosis. Unlike type 1 diabetes, which is not caused by diet and lifestyle but by an inflammatory destruction of the pancreas, type 2 diabetes is greatly affected by diet and lifestyle (and can often be treated, especially at the prediabetic stage, with diet and lifestyle changes). This important distinction means that by adaptation of an effective diet that brings blood sugar levels down, we may be able to prevent, slow down, or even potentially reverse type 2 diabetes.

Officially, type 2 diabetes is diagnosed through three tests: a fasting blood sugar test (your blood sugar when you wake up after not eating all night), a glucose tolerance test (a test of how your blood sugar reacts after drinking a pure glucose solution), and a hemoglobin A1c (HbA1c) test (a blood measure that is indicative of your average glucose levels over the past two to three months).

Once you have type 2 diabetes, there are several types of therapies that can help control your blood sugar. You could be prescribed various drugs (such as sulfonylurea) that encourage underperforming beta cells to produce more insulin. You could take other drugs (such as metformin and others) that encourage your liver and peripheral organs to uptake more sugar. And/or you can take injected insulin to supplement the reduced output from your exhausted pancreas. Some people with diabetes may not need insulin, but if the disease isn't managed, they probably will need it at some stage.

HbA1c: Your Blood Sugar over Time

HbA1c is a test that measures the percentage of your hemoglobin that is glycated, or that has a glucose molecule attached to it. A normal result would usually be at around 5 percent or less. Higher levels mean that too much of your hemoglobin is attached to sugar molecules. This test is interesting because, while a single test of blood sugar while fasting can only be predictive of a person's glucose levels at the time of measurement, the HbA1c test shows a longer-term picture: It represents your average blood sugar level over the past two to three months. If your blood sugar rises frequently and regularly, this will be reflected in your HbA1c percentage.

Several studies have associated abnormal HbA1c levels with a risk of developing cardiovascular disease, even in people without diabetes. One study showed that nondiabetics with HbA1c levels below 5 percent had low incidence of cardiovascular disease and mortality from any cause, but that every 1 percent increase above 5 percent was associated with a higher relative risk of death from any cause, even after correcting for other factors that could influence results, such as excessive weight, high blood pressure, high cholesterol levels, and cardiovascular disease history.[5] Another study showed that HbA1c levels could predict heart attacks in people with normal blood sugar levels.[6] For all these reasons, this is a useful test in analyzing blood sugar tendencies and diagnosing prediabetes or diabetes.

It is our opinion that these conditions exist along a spectrum. You are not normal and healthy one day and suddenly prediabetic or diabetic the next day. People slide gradually into these conditions over time, often over the course of years, and often without realizing it. They may or may not know they have become insulin resistant, or prediabetic. They may not know they have metabolic syndrome, and they often do not know they have full-blown diabetes. The exact test results doctors currently use to diagnose metabolic syndrome, prediabetes, and diabetes are, frankly, somewhat arbitrary. There are official ranges, but these are all stops along one road that leads to poor health, and they all have one common element: poor blood sugar control.

It may be disturbing to know that so many people go undiagnosed, but it's not surprising. You can't feel diabetes. If you are very overweight, your doctor might suspect it, and obesity is a risk factor for blood sugar control problems, but people with diabetes aren't always overweight, and all obese people don't have diabetes.

A doctor might give you a blood sugar test at your annual checkup if you ask for it, but that will probably only be a fasting blood sugar level, which may or may not tell you how successfully you are controlling your blood sugar on a day-to-day basis.

But there is a measure that may be even more indicative of blood sugar control problems—a measure that could predict whether you might be inclined to develop insulin resistance, metabolic syndrome, or prediabetes that progresses to type 2 diabetes. It is called the *postmeal blood sugar response*.

We've already mentioned the postmeal blood sugar response in this book, as it was part of our previous research. But now this measure is directly relevant to you. Research has confirmed that your blood sugar response following eating is directly related to your chances of not only developing diabetes but also heart disease, cancer, and other chronic diseases.[7,8,9] This "postprandial glucose response," or postmeal blood sugar response, may be an even more precise indicator, or an earlier indicator, of prediabetes or diabetes than fasting blood sugar, glucose tolerance tests, or HbA1c tests. And you can measure it for yourself. As you will see in the next chapter, this is a major focus of our personalized nutrition research. It will also be your focus, as you begin the program portion of this book, because how high your blood sugar goes after eating any given food is a direct measure of how harmful that food may be to your health. How often you eat those harmful foods can be indicative of your future diabetes risk.

Other Reasons to Control Your Blood Sugar

Diabetes isn't the only problem that can develop from poor blood sugar control and blood sugar that is too high. When your blood sugar remains too high for too long, or regularly goes too high after eating, you will also be at a higher risk for the following:

- **Weight gain and excess body fat.** Studies have shown that there is increased fat burning (fat oxidation) after eating meals that do not substantially raise glucose levels, while there is more fat storage after eating meals with high glucose responses, at least partially due to the anabolic effects exerted by insulin.[10] Research on rats shows that higher glucose responses after meals led to weight gain and that higher insulin responses (caused by high glucose responses) increased body fat.[11,12] In other words, if the foods you eat cause large spikes and dips in blood sugar, you are more likely to store fat and gain weight than if the foods you eat keep your blood sugar more even.

- **Hunger, food cravings, and low energy levels.** When blood sugar spikes trigger high insulin secretion, this may cause blood sugar to drop below a given person's blood sugar baseline (the level of blood sugar before eating, or upon first waking). This causes an intense feeling of hunger, especially for sugar or starch, which often results in subsequent overeating, continuing the unhealthy vicious eating-hunger-eating cycle. Many people also report intense feelings of fatigue and low energy with both blood sugar spikes and insulin spikes.

- **Overall mortality.** It may sound extreme to say that if your blood sugar goes up after meals, you are more likely to die. However, at least one study showed that higher blood sugar levels 1 hour after meals, even when they were still within "normal" range, was a good predictor of death from all causes for more than 2,000 healthy (nondiabetic) people during the thirty-three-year study.[13] The high blood sugar itself doesn't kill people, but it leads to or is associated with many other health consequences that may put you at greater risk for early death.

- **Heart disease.** We know high blood sugar in general contributes to heart disease. This has been well demonstrated in many studies. One study specifically showed a significant association between frequent high blood sugar levels after eating and cardiovascular events, as well as a generally higher tendency to die from any cause during the study's fourteen-year follow-up.[14] In other words, the study suggested that if you tend to have high blood sugar after eating, you are more likely to have a heart attack or die from any other cause!

Another study showed that high blood sugar 1 hour after a glucose challenge test (which simulates eating a meal) correlated with many different markers for heart disease, such as inflammation, abnormal lipid ratios, and insulin resistance, even in those who were not diabetic.[15] Yet another study showed that in nondiabetic, postmenopausal women, there was no association with fasting blood sugar levels and atherosclerosis (narrowing of the major arteries, including those supplying the heart, brain, and peripheral organs, which ultimately results in heart attack and stroke), but there was a *strong association* between high blood sugar levels after a glucose tolerance test and the progression of atherosclerosis, the underlying cause of ischemic heart disease and most cases of stroke.[16] Another study demonstrated that high blood sugar makes LDL cholesterol (the "bad" cholesterol) "stickier" and more likely to cling to the artery wall, increasing coronary heart disease risk—more evidence that abnormal blood sugar, and not just abnormal cholesterol, is a risk factor and that, in fact, they may work together to worsen cardiovascular health.[17]

These links to cardiovascular problems—and you can see there are many—are related to *postmeal blood sugar responses*, not just fasting glucose responses, diabetes diagnoses, or other typical blood-sugar-related risk factors.[18] *It is the postmeal glucose response that matters*, long before any disease diagnosis, and it is the exact same postmeal glucose response that can be controlled by the personalized diet. This is one of the reasons why we chose this measure for our research, as you will see in the next chapter, and why we also chose it for you to test on yourself, as you will see in "Part II: The Personalized Diet Program."

- **Cancer.** While we don't have any direct evidence that high blood glucose after meals causes cancer, there is some interesting research[19,20,21,22,23] suggesting that high postmeal blood glucose and high fasting glucose may be associated with enhanced risk of tumor progression. There is a phenomenon called the *Warburg effect* that was first discovered in 1924 by the German physiologist and Nobel laureate Otto Warburg. In one of his important discoveries, Warburg showed that cancer cells have a much different metabolism than regular cells. They rely heavily on sugar to survive and grow, metabolizing glucose at extremely high rates as compared to healthy cells. The idea that "sugar feeds cancer" has been out there for many years because of this research, but usually only in holistic health circles. When the genetics of cancer became a popular area of study, sugar as a key player in cancer fell out of favor, but cancer researchers have recently begun to focus on this phenomenon again. It is possible (although more research is required) that tumors really are more likely to thrive and grow in a glucose-rich environment[24,25] and that when glucose is in limited supply, tumor cell growth may be affected, but this is still a preliminary theory. We believe this is a promising area of research. There has also been some research associating high postmeal blood sugar with cancer, high fasting glucose with cancer, and a report showing that eliminating dietary carbohydrates can slow cancer progression. These associations merit further studies in humans.

- **Dementia.** Anyone with a family member suffering from dementia is likely to be highly motivated to avoid this degenerative brain issue. Managing blood sugar may be one powerful way to do this. There is a theory that blood vessel damage from frequent high blood sugar levels also includes damage to blood vessels in the brain. This damage could impede blood flow to the brain, worsening dementia symptoms. There are many studies showing that type 2 diabetes is a risk factor for dementia. Dementia and diabetes share several features, such as impaired glucose metabolism, insulin resistance, oxidative stress, and amyloidosis (the production of amyloid plaques in the brain, which are associated in some cases of elderly individuals with a risk of dementia),[26] and when the two disorders occur together, likely each condition makes the other worse.[27]

    Interestingly, at least one study showed that above-average blood sugar levels, even when they were not high enough to be considered diagnostic of diabetes, correlated to increased dementia risk.[28] Another disturbing study showed that blood sugar levels on the high end of the normal range in people without diabetes may be associated with a risk of cognitive impairment and increase the risk of brain shrinkage associated with aging and dementia—specifically, atrophy of the hippocampal region.[29] Perhaps blood sugar levels that are currently considered normal are actually too high.

- **Nerve damage.** Nerve damage is considered a common complication of long-term diabetes. However, even in people without diabetes, research suggests that nerve damage can occur when blood sugar stays elevated 2 hours after eating.[30] Another study showed that while diabetics had damage to large nerve fibers, nondiabetics (or prediabetics) with higher postmeal blood sugar had measurable damage to small nerve fibers.[31]

It's important to realize that your blood sugar level changes *mostly* in response to food, so what you eat is crucial for managing

Health associations of elevated postmeal blood sugar

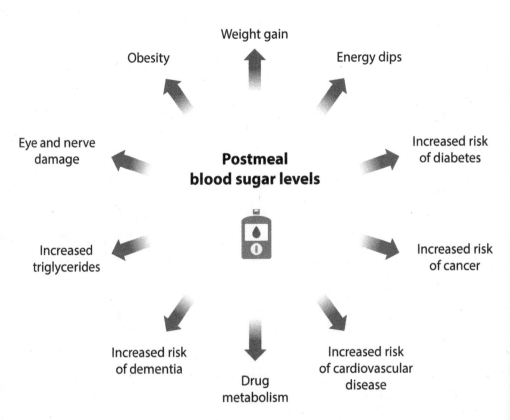

your blood sugar, and in turn, controlling your weight and regulating your health. Food choices are not only about calories and nutrients. If you eat to keep your blood sugar steady, you will lower your risk of obesity and metabolic disease, not to mention increase your energy and wakefulness.

The cause of your abnormal blood sugar levels might be simple—as simple as that sandwich you eat every day. Or, it may be more complex, the result of many different harmful food choices and habits. (This is what you will discover in Part II.)

The problem is, most people have no idea what their blood sugar levels are at any given time. The only reason Shay, our pilot study participant, found out that bread was spiking his blood sugar was because he was enrolled in our study. Fortunately, there is a way you *can* discover what your blood sugar is doing—and you don't have to be in a study to do so. We will explain how you can monitor your blood sugar with a simple device in Part II.

How to Improve Blood Sugar Control

But here's the good news: At any point during this dysfunctional slide from spikes in postmeal sugars to insulin resistance to actual diabetes, a dietary and lifestyle change that results in fewer glucose spikes and more normal glucose levels can help turn the damage around. What we choose to eat is the biggest factor in what our blood sugar does, so we can make different choices and influence our own blood sugar levels in a powerful way. The question is: What different choices should we make?

There are many theories about the best way to control blood sugar. We know exercise helps—specifically brief periods of high-intensity exercise,[32] but moderate-intensity exercise works as well.[33] We know a low-carbohydrate diet helps some people,[34,35] a low-fat diet seemed to help some,[36] a vegan diet proved helpful to some,[37] and a diet high in whole grains also seemed to help.[38] The American Diabetes Association recommends choosing foods that have a smaller impact on blood sugar,[39] and some research supports this.[40] Other research, however, suggests it doesn't actually help reduce the risk of diabetes or heart disease.[41] The fact that there is so much conflicting research on what actually helps blood sugar control is, in our estimation, further evidence that blood sugar control is a highly individual matter. Let's look more closely at one method that has received quite a lot of attention for its supposed ability to control blood sugar fluctuations: eating foods with a lower glycemic index (GI). Could this finally be an answer to blood sugar control for all?

How Lifestyle Influences Blood Sugar

Food may be the most obvious modifier of blood sugar levels, but other lifestyle choices that have nothing to do with your diet can also have a major impact on your blood sugar and ultimately your diabetes risk. Overall, just as with food, the lifestyle factors that can potentially influence your blood sugar levels in both directions are most likely to be variable:

- **High-intensity exercise.** During high-intensity exercise, your blood sugar levels will rise, because your body is breaking down glycogen so it can be used by your muscle cells. However, the short-term blood sugar rise is worth it because the beneficial effects, including increased insulin sensitivity (the opposite of insulin resistance, and your body's natural state) and improved glucose control, last for up to three days after exercise.

- **Sleep.** Research shows that sleep loss impairs glucose metabolism and raises insulin levels,[42] which in turn can lead to obesity and diabetes.
- **Stress.** Stress is linked to blood sugar surges, and high blood sugar, even among those who do not have diabetes, can cause severe health issues, especially in people who have experienced trauma or critical illness.[43] In some people, stress can also lead to blood sugar going too low.
- **Medications.** There are multiple medications known to increase blood sugar levels,[44] including birth control pills, progestin, niacin supplements, certain decongestants, barbiturates, corticosteroids, antipsychotics, and diuretics.[45] Other medications can cause blood sugar to go too low (hypoglycemia), including some antibiotics, beta blockers, and of course diabetes drugs like metformin and insulin.[46]
- **Smoking.** Smoking increases the risk of insulin resistance,[47] which can lead to elevated blood sugar levels.
- **Hormone fluctuations.** Some women who are menstruating experience higher blood sugar during that time of the month, but others don't.[48] This effect appears to be highly individual.
- **Fasting.** Going for long periods without eating can cause blood sugar to drop too low.[49]
- **Artificial sweeteners.** Our research shows that artificial sweeteners alter gut bacteria in a manner that can disrupt glucose metabolism in some people.[50]

It is clear from these factors that adaptation of a healthy lifestyle—sleeping enough, managing stress, quitting smoking, and avoiding artificial sweeteners—will increase your chances of maintaining stable blood sugar, even if you don't ever measure it, and is worth adapting and likely won't have a negative effect on your health. However, the best way to determine exactly what impacts your blood sugar and how to normalize it effectively over time can only be found through blood sugar testing.

THE GLYCEMIC INDEX

The GI is a system for ranking foods according to how much they influence blood sugar. It is based on a scale from 1 to 100. Foods with no carbohydrate content, such as olive oil or steak, do not have a GI because they don't contain any carbohydrates and should not therefore directly influence blood sugar. Pure glucose is ranked 100 because it should increase blood sugar (blood glucose) more than any other food. Every food containing carbohydrates is ranked somewhere between 1 and 100. This sounds sensible, especially because eating low-GI food is not only widely promoted in health literature but is also part of many popular diets. Theoretically, consumption of high-GI foods will cause a blood sugar spike, and consumption of low-GI foods will keep blood sugar more stable. If we can know for sure a food's likelihood of spiking or not spiking our blood sugar, we could finally know what to eat for maximum health benefits.

The problem is, the GI does not actually reveal this information. Most GI values you see in books or on the Web are based on an experiment conducted by one company (there is no official body that does this or sanctions the publication of GI values). For this experiment, a small group of people drank pure glucose and their blood sugar values were measured. Then they ate different foods, and their blood sugar values were recorded and averaged to come to a final number between 1 and 100.[51] So far, so good. But remember the limitation of only following averages. If everyone who ate a particular food, such as a banana, had very similar blood sugar responses, then the average could be considered a fairly reliable indicator for how most people will respond to that food. However, if the blood glucose responses to a food—say, an apple—varied widely, with some people experiencing a very high response to apples while others experience a very low response to the same apples, then the average of those responses will not be informative to any of these tested people. You would never know if you were a very high or a very low responder to that food from the GI, which would be a value in the middle.

For example, the following figure shows the responses of a group of people who were tested for their blood sugar responses to both bananas and apples. The responses to bananas were quite similar. An average of these numbers, all cluttered around 65, is likely to be accurate for most people. However, the responses to apples range from about 45 all the way up to nearly 90. An average for an apple would also be 65, the same as for a banana. But the individual response to an apple could be anywhere in the rage of 45 to 90 (and possibly outside of either of those results). It's likely that you would respond to a banana like others in the study, but not so with the apple. Going by the GI, you would never know for sure whether apples were giving you a blood sugar spike or were a good choice for you, personally. Therefore, knowing the GI value of a banana might be helpful for you, but knowing the GI value of an apple probably would not. The GI index itself cannot tell you which values will match your reactions to any food.

Two foods with the same glycemic index (averaged across people) but very different behaviors across individuals

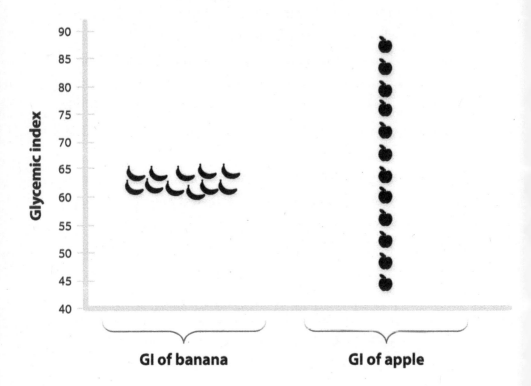

GI of banana   **GI of apple**

There are some additional problems with GI values:

- The GI can be used only for foods and meals for which it has been measured. You cannot extrapolate the GI of an unmeasured food based on the GI of existing measured foods.

- The GI is not additive, meaning that you cannot measure the GI of, for example, broccoli, add it to the GI of carrots, and know for sure how a meal containing broccoli and carrots will behave together. Because people don't usually eat single foods alone, any food combining may render the GI values of the individual foods meaningless.

- You cannot know the impact of adding additional ingredients into the meal, which may not have been measured. Broccoli and carrots in a homemade cream or cheese sauce will be an unknown quantity.
- GI is also used to evaluate glycemic load (GL) and measures the relationship between carbohydrate content in a certain food and the amount of carbohydrate in a serving size of that food. For example, if the GI of a baked potato is 111, the GL of a 5-ounce baked potato is 33. It is difficult to try to figure out what these different numbers mean, and you cannot determine what will happen to these numbers if you add butter and sour cream to your baked potato, or if your baked potato weighs 8 ounces instead of 5 ounces. And without considering the GL, the influence of blood sugar isn't linear. There is no way to determine how the GI will change according to your portion size.
- Using GI can be problematic, and research into the effectiveness of eating according to the GI confirms this. Some studies show that a diet high in high-GI foods is associated with a higher risk of diabetes and cardiovascular disease, while others show no association at all. All this throws into question the benefit of using the GI to find the right foods to lower blood sugar. Because the research on the effectiveness of the GI is so varied, this is just another reason why knowing your own blood sugar responses is the only real way to make food choices that you know will keep your blood sugar stable. If you were not one of the people in the experiment used to create the GI, you will never know what your own blood sugar values will be

after eating a food. In fact, your response may be quite different, and even opposite from those measured people, whose responses were all averaged anyway. The GI may have nothing to do with you as an individual.

Your blood sugar responses are unique, and while they may correspond to standard measurements like the glycemic index some of the time, this will not always be true. You cannot be sure whether your blood sugar will become unstable with over-eating, or with a consistent high-carb or high-fat diet. You cannot be sure that any blood sugar "rules" derived from anyone else will apply to you.

CARB COUNTING

A simpler way that many people try to figure out how to control their blood sugar—and a method often recommended by doctors for their diabetic patients—is to count carb grams. Anyone who has ever tried a low-carb diet is probably familiar with this idea. Because higher-carbohydrate meals usually (on average) induce higher postmeal blood glucose levels, counting carbohydrates sounds like a rational approach for assessing postmeal blood sugar rise.

We saw this result in the study we will tell you about in the next chapter—of the approximately 50,000 meals consumed by our study participants, we found a significant association between the carb content and the postmeal blood sugar response. However, there were many exceptions—people who had a high blood sugar response to meals with a low carbohydrate content and people who had a low blood sugar response from a meal containing a high carbohydrate content. Just because a majority reacted with a high postmeal blood sugar response to a high-carb meal does not mean that everyone did, and in fact, many did not. So as with the GI, carb counting *might* be indicative of how you will respond to a food but will not tell you for sure whether rice or bread or cookies or ice cream are creating unhealthy blood sugar spikes for you.

Other research has shown that carbohydrate counting doesn't work very well.[52] The reasons for this are twofold:

1. As we saw in our study, people have different sensitivities to carbs. Some people respond very strongly, others do not, so a single value for a given amount of carbs predicting the response for all people would not work.
2. Meals are complex. Some have more fat or protein, which tends to blunt postmeal blood sugar (but not always). Context also matters. If meals are eaten before or after exercise or at different times of day, these factors also have an effect— that is, two meals that are identical in calories but that vary in fat or protein, proximity to exercise, or time of day have been shown to have quite variable blood sugar responses in different people. For these reasons, a model using only carb content will not be a good predictor of response.

Carb Counting for Diabetics

People with type 1 diabetes who lose their beta cells because of pancreatic inflammation and are dependent on injected insulin are often instructed to count their carbs to help them determine the insulin dosage they need to inject after meals to keep their

glucose levels intact, but it is well known in the scientific literature that this approach doesn't work very well. Patients often
report that when they base their dosage on carb counting, they
sometimes do not inject enough insulin, and then their blood
sugar levels remain too high after meals, or they inject too much
insulin and go into a dangerous hypoglycemic state, requiring
more sugar to raise their blood sugar to a safe level. This often
becomes a vicious cycle.

We have a mutual friend who has type 1 diabetes who
describes this exact problem. He told us that it is very hard for
him to predict his blood sugar levels based on carb counting and
that his levels sometimes depend on the time of day, whether he
exercised the day before, and other factors having nothing to do
with the carbohydrate content of his meals. This is very frustrating for him because it is a daily chore, constantly estimating his
responses to control his glucose level. One long-term goal of our
research is to reveal a better, more accurate, and therefore safer
method for people with diabetes to determine what their insulin
dosages should be. In fact, we are currently performing research
on this exciting new concept, with both juvenile (type 1) and
adult-onset (type 2) diabetes.

But there is something you can discover that can influence
your weight, your energy, and your health risks. You can determine your unique blood sugar response to a meal you just ate, in
real time. You can measure your blood sugar and get immediate
information about the effect of the food you just ate. Unlike trying to find a GI list on the Internet and hoping it will tell you
something useful, blood sugar is an easy way to measure, is accurate, and reveals an individual response to eating particular foods.

We chose blood sugar as the crux of our research and used
it as the primary measure that helped us determine, for each

individual, exactly what foods result in a positive blood sugar response and what foods result in dangerous blood sugar spikes. It was a fascinating, surprising, illuminating, and paradigm-shifting experiment that demonstrated how much individual people can learn about how to eat in a personalized way, as well as what happens when they design a personalized diet based on those blood sugar results.

CHAPTER 7

The Personalized Nutrition Project

Donna and her family originally came from the United States, but they have been living in Israel for a few years. Before they relocated, they believed that changing their diets from the standard American diet to the "Mediterranean diet" would benefit everyone in the family. They had heard about the healthful way people supposedly eat in this region of the world. Instead, however, after living in Israel for a while, the whole family gained weight. Donna and her husband, Charles, were concerned. Why were they gaining weight in an environment with such healthful food choices? Why were their children gaining weight? They wanted to participate in the Personalized Nutrition Project, not only so they could contribute to science but also so they could learn something about themselves. They didn't imagine it would change their lives.

Donna and Charles signed up for our study and began tracking their blood sugar responses to foods. The first thing they discovered related to hamburgers. Hamburgers were a favorite family meal they always served with a side of guilt, thinking they were "junk food." They were quite surprised to learn that this family favorite resulted in perfectly healthy blood sugar responses for both of them. However, many of the foods the family consumed heavily, like cereal, pita bread, and rice, spiked both Donna's and Charles's blood sugar to abnormal levels. While they had some different responses to foods, they also found multiple foods that were good for both of them—often not the foods they expected. After the study, they shaped the family diet around their mutual "good" foods and away from their mutual "bad" foods. Although the children had not been tested (the study included only people aged eighteen and over), they hoped that since they had so many common measures, their children were likely to respond in a similar way. Just as they had hoped, everyone in the family gradually began to lose weight, including the children. Everybody also noticed they had more energy. The oldest child joined a local soccer team, and Donna and Charles quickly realized (and told their friends) that they had finally found a rational way to turn around the whole family's health and energy that was compatible with everyone's life and preferences.

Having an individual response to foods makes sense on an intuitive level. We know we are all different. We know we each have different genetics and different lifestyles, and in recent years, we have learned that we all have different compositions of gut bacteria. These factors translate to having different enzymes, different genes, different bacterial genes, and probably many other unique factors that have yet to be discovered. It's no wonder we all respond differently to the same foods. It's no wonder diets and dietary recommendations intended for everyone don't work for everyone. It's almost as if this should have been our initial assumption: that different people would respond differently to, say, a slice of bread or a cookie or a T-bone steak; to a hamburger or a bowl of cereal. If we all responded the same way, that would be the surprising result.

It also makes sense, even without any science to back it up, that a universal diet would not be equally effective for everyone. Yet, this hadn't really been proven in a way that satisfies people. It has also not been the current practice or thinking of governmental agencies and policy makers seeking to offer advice and guidance on diet.

We want to change that thinking. Our own research, performed on an unprecedented number of more than 1,000 research subjects, has effectively demonstrated exactly why nutrition, to be most beneficial to any individual human being, absolutely must be personalized.

SETTING UP THE STUDY

We knew we needed a new approach to understand and hopefully predict postmeal blood sugar response in individuals. We also knew from the failures of the glycemic index that averages across groups of people are not sufficiently informative for any one person trying to get control of blood sugar. Our first goal was to prove that different people respond to foods differently, even the same foods in the same amounts. As we've already discussed, we chose blood sugar as a primary measure, because:

- postmeal blood sugar provides an immediate, measurable response to food;
- blood sugar fluctuation is a good marker for weight and health issues;
- blood sugar monitoring has good technology—we could measure blood sugar in our study subjects every 5 minutes for an entire week, resulting in glucose responses for approximately 50,000 meals and snacks overall.

We began by enlisting 1,000 healthy volunteers to participate in our study. We were pleased to find out that people were eager to sign up, saying they wanted to learn more about themselves, get personalized information about what to eat, know what their microbiome contained, and/or lose weight.

The people who joined our study ranged in age between eighteen and seventy and had not been diagnosed with adult-onset diabetes (this was a requirement of participation because we wanted to study blood sugar responses in healthy, nondiabetic people). About half of the participants were overweight and about a quarter of them were obese, approximating the adult nondiabetic population in Israel where we did the study, in the United States, and in the developed world generally.

First, we collected a lot of information about each person— how often they ate, how they lived, and their medical backgrounds. We took body measurements like height, weight, and hip circumference. We did a panel of blood tests and took a stool sample from each person to profile their microbiome.

Why Include the Microbiome?

Of all the measures in our study, gut bacteria was perhaps the most novel and curious factor we examined. Nobody else studying blood sugar has done this, so why did we include it? As discussed in Chapter 5, and as scientists are now just learning, the microbiome has a major effect on weight, health, and blood sugar responses. We also know from our research that everyone has a unique microbiome "signature," so we wanted to discover whether that unique signature had anything to do with unique blood sugar responses. Our previous research into the microbiome has proven to be illuminating, so we felt it was necessary to discover whether the microbiome was a major player in personalized nutrition. As you will see in this chapter, it was.

Next, we connected each participant to a glucose sensor and tracked his/her blood glucose levels continuously for a full week (right now, this technology is only available by prescription for people with a diabetes diagnosis, but we will approximate this technology using blood sugar meters, in the next section). During that week, participants logged everything they ate on a mobile app we developed—an app we have also personalized for use by the readers of this book. While we let our study participants eat what they would normally eat for most meals, we wanted to have one meal standardized between all the different participants, so we always provided everyone with breakfast consisting of a rotating menu of plain bread, bread with butter, fructose powder mixed with water, or glucose powder mixed with water. Not a particularly delicious or hearty breakfast, we admit, but this allowed us to accurately compare various responses to uniform meals across our study population. Altogether, we were able to gather data on nearly 7,000 separate breakfasts, as well as 50 distinct meals per participant, totaling around 50,000 meals across all 1,000 people, with 10 million calories logged, along with huge amounts of associated health data.

The result of these parameters was that we had an unprecedented amount of very specific data to work with—and this also made ours the largest study by far ever to focus on postmeal blood sugar response.

In the second phase of the study, we took this massive amount of data and used it to create an algorithm that could predict, even in someone who was not part of the original study, exactly what their postmeal blood sugar response would be to most foods, based on a few simple health measures and a microbiome sample.

What We Discovered

After all the data came rolling in and we analyzed it, we realized we had stumbled across a shocking realization: *Everything was personal.* In other words, for every single medical or nutritional finding that came up in this study, there were *many people whose results were very different from it.* For example, for every food that was likely to cause a high postmeal blood sugar response on average (such as pita bread), there were people who had a low postmeal blood sugar response to it, and for every food that was likely to cause a low postmeal blood sugar response on average (like chocolate, probably due to its high fat content), there were those people who had a high postmeal blood sugar response to it.

In the following figure, you can see that different foods have different averages. For example, chocolate and ice cream have low average postmeal blood sugar responses, but the bars show the *actual* (not averaged) variations across people in the study. You can see here that for meals with high average postmeal blood sugar responses, there are also those who responded even lower than those who responded to meals with low averages.

Before we get too much into the variability and personalization aspect of our study, let's first discuss the significant non-personalized trends our study uncovered. A word of caution: While these are *general* trends, and your individual response

Average blood glucose responses to different foods in our study

Sorting is by the average response. Bars represent percentiles 25–75.
Note that for each food there is high variability across people in the blood glucose response.

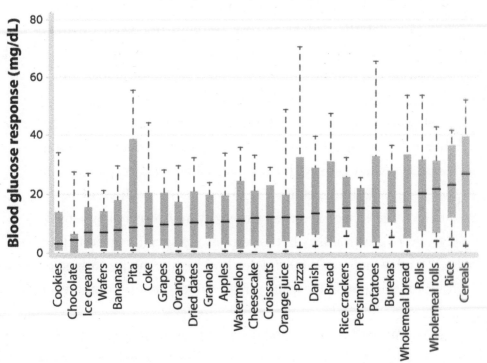

may be different from the majority, you are *likely* to have similar responses. Blood sugar testing can confirm this, but before you try, here are some things to consider about what affected blood sugar fluctuations in many, and sometimes most, of our study participants. The first four trends we describe in the following pages are related to food, but the remaining trends were related to the person eating it.

Generalized Trend #1: Carbohydrate Content

As we mentioned in the previous chapter, we saw a trend of carbohydrate amount significantly correlating with postmeal blood sugar response. The more carbs, generally, the higher the response. Many people in the study were quite carb-sensitive, meaning that their meal glucose response followed carb content quite closely. These people would probably benefit, in general, from carb counting, or even from following the GI, in the absence of more specific information.

However, we also found many people who were not carb-sensitive, and for those people, carb content in the food had little or no association with postmeal blood sugar response. This was surprising but certain. There was also a gradient of people between these two extremes, from very high to very low sensitivity, as well as variability in the response to specific carbohydrate-rich foods (such as a high/low or low/high response to fructose solution compared to white bread or ice cream compared to cookies).

Overall, carb counting alone *could not reliably predict* postmeal blood sugar response in any one individual, but the correlation was there, in general.

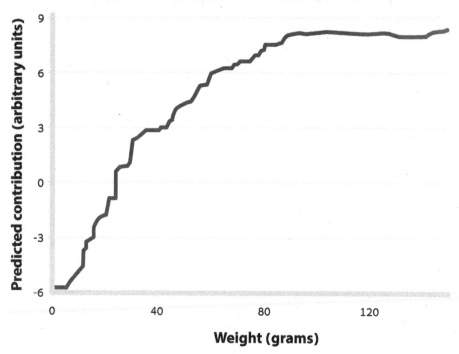

Carbohydrate trend: Higher carbohydrates in the meal are associated, on average, with a higher glucose response.

Generalized Trend #2: Fat Content

In general, the more fat added to a meal, the lower the postmeal blood sugar response. This may sound surprising but is actually consistent with previous studies that have shown that adding fat to meals can reduce the postmeal blood sugar response.[1] But here, too, we found that this effect varied according to the person and was therefore not a collectively reliable strategy. Many people in the study had a reduced postmeal blood sugar response with the addition of fat, but for others, this had little to no effect. If you discover that you get a blood sugar spike from eating a high-carb food such as bread, you might be able to correct this by simply adding some fat, such as butter.

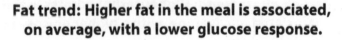

Fat trend: Higher fat in the meal is associated, on average, with a lower glucose response.

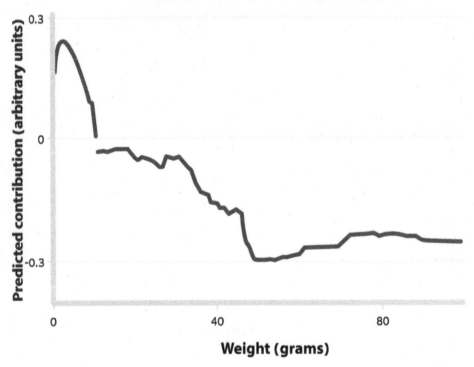

Weight (grams)

Generalized Trend #3: Fiber Content

The trend regarding fiber was interesting in a complex way. In general, higher fiber within a meal tended to increase postmeal blood sugar response for that meal but had a longer-term positive lower sugar spike effect *in future meals*. In other words, 24 hours after eating a high-fiber meal, most people's blood sugar response improved even when the fiber-containing meal had a higher postmeal blood sugar response at the time.

Because we digest dietary fiber solely through the action of our gut bacteria, we suspect that this positive effect of delayed, reduced postmeal blood sugar response may be due to a slight shift in gut bacteria responding to the added fiber.

However, while we found many people who had a short-term adverse effect from fiber and a long-term beneficial effect from fiber, it may also be true that some people have both a short-term and a long-term positive effect from fiber. Others might have a short-term and long-term negative effect from fiber. This is what we would expect, considering the evidence we have found for personalization, but this area needs more research. As for you, in Part II, you will get the opportunity to discover whether you have a positive or negative response to high-fiber foods.

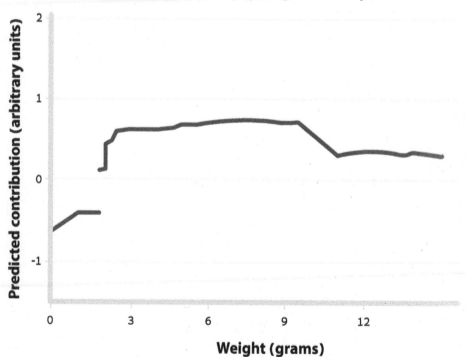

Fiber trend: Higher fiber content in the meal is associated, on average, with a higher glucose response.

Generalized Trend #4: Sodium and Water Content

In general, a higher sodium content in food was associated with a higher postmeal blood sugar response, but a higher water content was associated with a lower postmeal blood sugar response. There is evidence, as discussed earlier in this book, that limiting salt in the diet is probably unnecessary for most people. Our current study suggests that in some cases, and for some people, salt may have a negative effect on postmeal blood sugar response, but not necessarily in everyone. In some participants, sodium did not increase postmeal blood sugar response.

Sodium content of meal

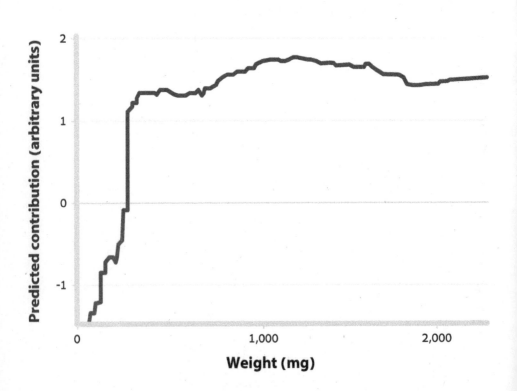

Weight (mg)

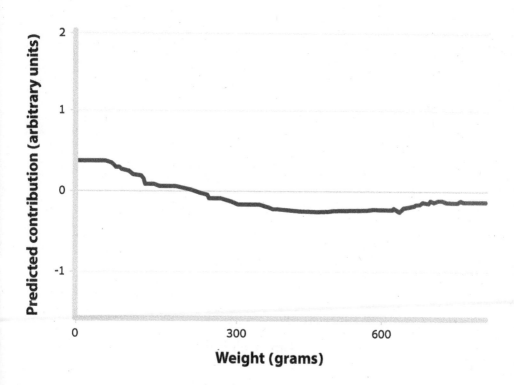

Water content of meal

Generalized Trend #5: Timing of Meals in Relation to Waking

The more time that had elapsed from waking, the higher the postmeal blood sugar response, so the breakfast postmeal blood sugar response was generally lower than the blood sugar response after dinner. This was not true for everyone, however. Some participants experienced the exact opposite—their highest blood sugar responses occurred during the morning and were higher at breakfast than at dinner. When you test your own blood sugar in Part II, you will have the opportunity to discover whether

Time from waking

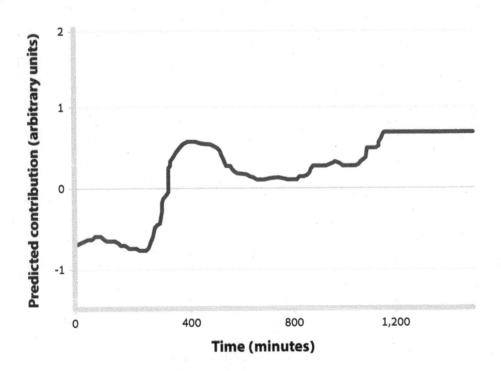

you are more likely to have higher blood sugar responses in the morning or the evening.

Generalized Trend #6: Health Risk Factors

When it came to risk factors, our data revealed some striking trends. Postmeal blood sugar responses were generally higher in the presence of several known health risk factors, including the following:

- **BMI.** This measurement of body fat is based on weight in relation to height (there are many BMI calculators available online that can help you determine yours, if you don't already know it).[2] Our study clearly showed that the

Higher blood glucose responses are associated with higher BMI.

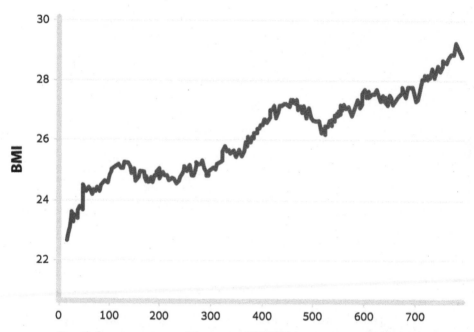

Participants, sorted by meal PPGR (postprandial glucose response, i.e., glucose response after eating)

higher your BMI, the more likely you are to experience higher-than-average postmeal blood sugar responses.

However, the correlation between BMI and postmeal blood sugar response was not always true. Some people with high BMIs tended to have lower postmeal blood sugar responses, and some people with low BMIs tended to have higher ones.

- **HbA1c.** In the previous chapter, we talked about this measurement of blood sugar that reflects the levels over the past three months. This is one of the diagnostic tests for diabetes or prediabetes. Normal levels are between 4 percent

Higher blood glucose responses are associated with higher HbA1c%.

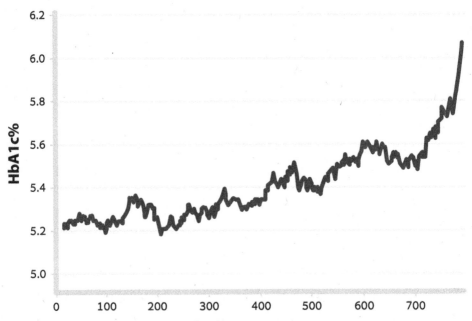

and 5.7 percent, but those with diabetes try to keep their levels under 7 percent.[3] In our study, in general, the higher the HbA1c percentage, the higher the likelihood of elevated postmeal blood sugar responses. As always, there were exceptions.

- **Fasting glucose.** This test of blood sugar first thing in the morning is a primary test for diabetes. Normal levels are typically between 70 and 99 mg/dL (3.8 to 5.5 mmol). You are considered to have prediabetes if your fasting blood sugar is consistently 101 to 125 mg/dL (5.6 to 6.9 mmol), and you will be diagnosed with diabetes if your

Higher blood glucose responses are associated with higher fasting glucose levels.

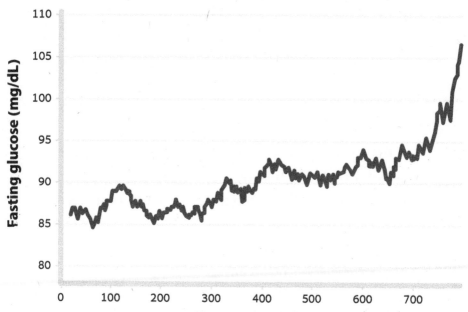

fasting blood sugar is consistently 126 mg/dL (7 mmol) or higher.[4] In our study, we saw a strong correlation between fasting glucose and postmeal blood sugar response—although as with all other measures, this did not apply to all participants.

- **Systolic blood pressure.** This is the top or first number in a standard blood pressure reading; the lower value is called the *diastolic blood pressure* and is equally important to many aspects of health. A systolic blood pressure of under 120 is considered normal. The higher the systolic blood pressure, the higher the postmeal blood sugar response in many people. (We also tested diastolic, but the correlation didn't appear to be significant.)

- **ALT, or alanine aminotransferase, activity.** These are typically measured (via a blood test) to help determine the health of your liver. Higher levels (correlated with liver damage) were often but not always correlated with higher postmeal blood sugar response. Higher ALT levels may indicate that you are developing fatty liver, a condition that is often found in obese or diabetic individuals.

- **CRP, or C-reactive protein.** This measure of inflammation somewhere in the body is considered a nonspecific marker of disease or infection and is correlated positively with postmeal blood sugar response in general, but not always.

- **Age.** We can't control this one, of course, but we did see a correlation between age and postmeal blood sugar response. The older you are, the more likely your postmeal blood sugar response will be elevated—but again, this was not always the case.

Interestingly, not all of the aforementioned trends were restricted to the extremes. For example, we did not see elevated postmeal blood sugar responses only in those with morbid obesity or diabetes-level HbA1c. Even within the normal range for BMI, those with higher numbers (such as 24 versus 22) tended to have higher postmeal blood sugar responses. This suggests that you don't have to have a serious level of risk factor for your blood sugar response to be affected. It seems to be influenced, *in general*, on a continuum throughout the entire range of healthy to ill.

Generalized Trend #7: Microbiome

Most people don't know their own microbiome composition. This kind of testing for the consumer is very new and only recently becoming available (see page 305 for more information on DayTwo, a company we consult and whose microbiome testing is based on our research). But someday soon, you probably will be able to discover your microbiome composition. When we tested those of our study participants, we saw many interesting trends related to specific bacteria in the microbiome. For example, having higher levels of a bacterium called *Parabacteroides distasonis* was associated with higher postmeal blood sugar responses, whereas higher levels of the bacteria *Bacteroides dorei* was associated with lower postmeal blood sugar responses.

Some bacteria have already been correlated with poor blood sugar control, as well as risk factors like obesity, insulin resistance, and impaired lipid profiles (such as high cholesterol).[5] These known correspondences generally applied in our study. For example, *Eubacterium rectale,* a bacteria that can ferment dietary carbohydrates and fibers to produce metabolites useful to you,[6] usually showed an association with lower postmeal blood sugar responses. Bacteria known to be associated with obesity, such as the aforementioned *Parabacteroides distasonis*[7] and *Bacteroides thetaiotaomicron,*[8] generally correlated with higher postmeal blood sugar response.

Also, the presence of certain bacteria was more likely to result in higher postmeal blood sugar responses for particular foods, such as white bread or fructose, but not for other foods. There were many more complex interactions involving the gut microbiota, some corresponding to standard beliefs about the beneficial or nonbeneficial nature of specific bacteria and others being novel findings about bacteria for which there were no previously known associations. The more we learn about the microbiome, the more this line of research will, we suspect, become particularly illuminating.

Generalized Trend #8: Outliers

As you've seen throughout this chapter, and as we hypothesized, there were outliers to every trend. No matter what was sometimes or often true, there were always people who did not respond as expected or who did not respond like the majority. The responses varied, not just according to the trends like weight or blood pressure, high carb or high sodium, but to very particular foods, like bananas and cookies. For example, the following two graphs show two different participants and their reactions to glucose solution versus bread and bananas versus cookies. Note how they have opposite responses to these high-carbohydrate foods. In one participant, cookies did not raise blood sugar but bananas did. In the other participant, it was the exact opposite.

These opposite reactions are the most interesting part of our study. Because our data set was so large and our analysis so comprehensive, these results have an enormous impact—they show more conclusively than has ever been shown before that a generic, universal approach to nutrition simply cannot work. This convinces us that food responses are highly personal and beyond any one measure (i.e., carbs, sugar, fat) and that diets that will maintain healthy blood glucose levels must therefore be personally tailored. It also explains, in our view, why the current

Example of two participants in our study who had opposite blood glucose responses to glucose and bread

(the top participant responded more highly to glucose, the lower to bread)

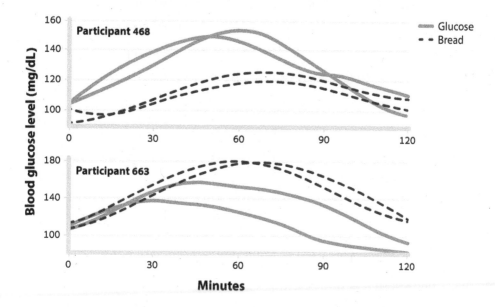

Example of two participants in our study who had opposite blood glucose responses to bananas and cookies

(the top participant responded more highly to banana, the lower to cookies)

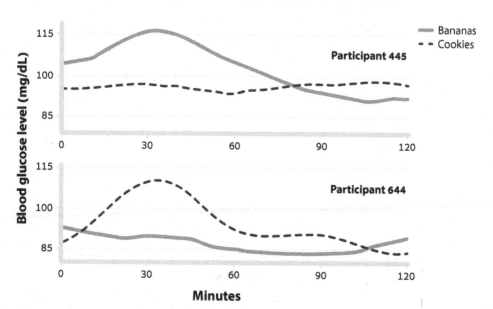

nutritional paradigm, which searches for that one best diet, is inherently flawed. The best diet for all people does not exist. Our response to food is personal, so our dietary advice must also be personal. But this was not the end of our research.

Eran Segal's Story: Eat Ice Cream, Not Rice?

Keren, my wife, is a clinical dietitian, and when I showed her the data from our study, the results shocked her. One example that struck her was our finding that some people had a postmeal blood sugar response spike after eating ice cream but not after eating rice, but that others—completely unexpectedly to her—spiked for rice (even brown rice) but not for ice cream. In fact, we found that *more people spiked for rice than for ice cream.*

As a dietitian, my wife relies on general dietary guidelines because this is how she was trained. Therefore, one of the first things she tells the many newly diagnosed prediabetics that she treats is to stop eating foods such as ice cream and instead eat more complex carbohydrates such as brown rice.

When she saw our data, she realized that for most of her patients, not only was her dietary advice unhelpful, but in fact, her advice could be pushing them more quickly toward the very disease her advice was meant to prevent! Now she advises her clients based on the trends we saw and advises them to test their own blood sugar responses to meals to see what foods are best for them.

Creating the Algorithm

Once we had all our data, the next step was to determine if we could translate it into useful information, especially if it was so variable and so resistant to obvious and universal patterns. The answer, we decided, was to try to put it all into an algorithm, a single complex formula, that a computer could use to predict, based on information about an individual (the information we collected at the beginning of our study, including the blood tests and microbiome sample), exactly what foods would be most likely to increase postmeal blood sugar response in any given person.

To develop this algorithm, we took the microbiome information and all other clinical data that we collected and devised advanced subalgorithms to automatically search for rules that predict personalized meal glucose responses. For example, if you are over fifty years old and have a certain species of bacteria, then your glucose response to a banana will be high. Then we plugged all that data into a super-algorithm that combined tens of thousands of such rules automatically deduced from the data. As you can see from the following two graphs, our algorithm was able to predict postmeal blood sugar response with much greater accuracy than carbohydrate counting.

Our algorithmic approach is similar to how websites like Amazon recommend books for you, except that we applied it to how people respond to food, and the result was a success. We took 100 new people who had not been part of our study and tried the algorithm on them. We worked very hard to reach this point—it was a major test for us, and we were eager to see the results. It was therefore a thrill to see that our algorithm could take any person, even people who were not part of the original study, and predict their personalized glucose response to any meal with high accuracy. It proved that our algorithm learned rules by which personal parameters associate with personalized meal glucose responses.

Meal carbohydrates is a significant but poor predictor of blood glucose response.

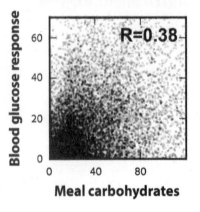

Our machine learning algorithm accurately predicts personalized blood glucose responses.

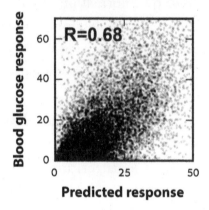

Having an algorithm that predicts personalized food responses motivated us to ask: Could our algorithm help to design personalized diets that would normalize blood glucose levels for anyone?

As a final step, we recruited and profiled twenty-six new participants, mostly prediabetics (who are interesting to us because their condition is quite common and can be reversed with the right diet). We asked the algorithm to design two diets for each person. In one diet, which we called the bad diet, we asked the algorithm to predict meals that would spike the person's glucose levels. In the other, the good diet, we asked it to predict meals for which that person would have low responses.

The participants then followed each of the diets for one week. We placed one restriction on the diets: All breakfasts, lunches, dinners, and snacks were identical in calories, whether on the good or bad diets. Each person received a different personalized diet based on the algorithm's predictions—it is interesting to note that there were foods on the good diet of some people that were on the bad diet of others.

Below are the two diets for one of our participants. You can see that the food choices are not those found in typical diets.

	Diet 1	*Diet 2*
Breakfast	Muesli	Eggs and bread
Lunch	Sushi	Hummus and pita
Afternoon Snack	Marzipan candy	Edamame
Dinner	Corn and nuts	Vegetable noodles with tofu
Night snack	Chocolate and coffee	Ice cream

Can you guess which one the algorithm predicted to be the good diet and the bad diet? As you can see, each diet contains foods such as ice cream and chocolate that would not typically appear in standard diets, as well as foods usually considered healthful, like sushi and nuts, or hummus and tofu.

We asked our students, who were not involved in this project, to guess which diet was which, and they were split nearly fifty-fifty. We have now given a lecture on this topic dozens of times, often to very large crowds, and when we ask this question, there is always a split, often around fifty-fifty. The question is not trivial, and the answer is not obvious. Neither of the diets looks conventional, and for a different subject in the study, the "good" and "bad" diet would be completely different. It's a puzzle that only the algorithm can answer.

In this case, Diet 2 was the diet predicted by the algorithm to be good for this participant, and Diet 1 was the diet predicted by the algorithm to be bad. For another participant, it may have been exactly the opposite.

Now that the algorithm could create good and bad diets, we were eager to see how well they worked in real life. We put information for each of our twenty-six new participants into the algorithm and created a good and a bad diet for each of them—fifty-two diets in total. They each followed their personalized good diet for one week and their personalized bad diet for the next week.

The following graph represents the glucose responses of the person given the good and bad diets shown in the preceding chart. This graph shows the continuous glucose levels of this participant during the bad diet (in black line) for an entire week and the good diet (the gray line) for an entire week. On the bad diet, you can clearly see abnormally high glucose levels after meals, indicating that this participant has impaired glucose metabolism and is probably prediabetic. This was the result while that participant was eating muesli, sushi, and nuts.

But on the good diet, which includes the eggs, noodles, and ice cream, and which *had the same number of calories in each meal as the bad diet*, the postmeal glucose levels remained fully normal, without a single spike across the entire week. We believe that if this participant followed this good diet (ice cream and all) for several more weeks, he may reverse his prediabetic state.

We found similar results in most participants for which we designed personally tailored good and bad diets using our algorithm. These results were frankly stunning to us—the proof that you can manipulate your own blood sugar levels so significantly that you can go from prediabetic blood sugar levels to normal

Comparison of the weeklong continuous blood glucose levels of one of the prediabetic participants who followed our "bad" diet (graph with spikes) and "good" diet (flat graph). Both diets had the same number of calories in each meal.

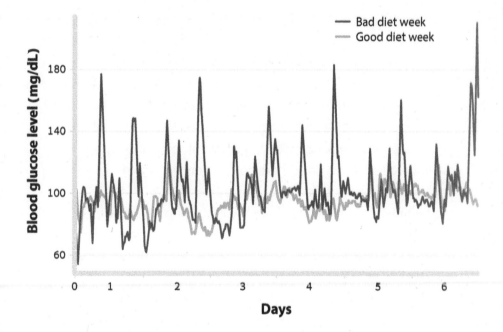

blood sugar levels in just one week, and only by changing your food choices, is unprecedented.

Sue C.

I am in my midforties and I work at an international corporate firm, so I travel frequently on transatlantic flights. For my entire life, I have been healthy. I smoke a little but I take no medications. I get annual physicals and have always had normal results on all tests. I'm mildly overweight, I admit, but I'm so busy that I don't really have time for any sort of formal weight management program or exercise routine.

When I heard about the Personalized Nutrition Project from a family friend who is a staff member for the researchers, after some persuasion, I agreed to enroll. I got some interesting dietary results, but the most important thing that came of it all was that I found out I have prediabetes! I had no idea I had this condition, but now I know that it affects almost 40 percent of the population. In my case, fasting blood sugar tests at the doctor during my annual physicals were not enough to discover I had this condition, but since I got measured continuously for an entire week during the study, my disturbed blood sugar responses were much more obvious and clearly above normal. I'm feeling very lucky with this diagnosis, as I now know that 70 percent of unmonitored people with prediabetes go on to develop full diabetes within a decade or two, and I do not plan to be one of them.

I made a complete shift in how I live. I stopped smoking out of concern for my heart. I stopped traveling across time zones so frequently, traveling only when necessary, and I also recognized that changing when I eat makes a real difference for my blood sugar control. I also changed my diet, of course. I eat less rice, avoid oranges, but can have a drink of beer once a week and have put my beloved cereal back on the menu. I even enrolled in a follow-up study for prediabetes, where I ate my personalized "Good" and "Bad" diets, each for a week, and amazingly, when I ate the "Good" diet personalized for me, my blood sugar levels became totally normal! I now follow that new diet and try to exercise more, and I'm feeling great! I am indebted to the Personalized Nutrition Project for my timely diagnosis and my ability to regain control over my health.

WHAT THIS MEANS FOR YOU

These results suggest many complex things and provide much hope for the future. Based on the large variability that we observed in the response to foods across 1,000 people, our conclusion is that *there is no one diet that is best for everyone.* If you have been suffering through diets that don't work, you can finally stop. We are simply all too different—and we now have conclusive proof. This means that if a certain diet hasn't worked for you, then it may have been the wrong diet for you. Your past diet "failures" may not be your fault. A diet may have failed simply because it did not take information about *you* as an individual into account.

The next step for us in our research is to start longer-term dietary intervention studies in both prediabetic and diabetic populations. These studies will last for a full year. Because we believe that the effect of normalizing blood sugar levels will persist for a longer period than the one week we have already observed, our hope is that a longer-term intervention could reverse and possibly cure the metabolic diseases that constitute one of the worst epidemics of our time. We believe that we now have the right approach and the right tools to do that, and that it can be done without drugs, simply by dietary changes customized to the individual.

More broadly, we believe that we are entering a new era in the study of nutrition. We believe that we are moving away from standardized diets and dietary advice and toward a frontier of personalization, in its many guises. We are learning to ask more targeted questions and we are finding out the answers. Someday, when your children or grandchildren are in school, we predict that they will not be given a lesson on nutritional guidelines that are one-size-fits-all. Instead, they may get a lesson on how to determine what nutritional guidelines are best for each individual. We look forward to that day.

And now you also have something to do. You can get in the game, too, by testing your own blood sugar and logging your results on our free app to determine what foods will stabilize *your* blood sugar. This could be exactly what it takes for you to finally drop excess weight, gain energy, and get healthy. The next chapter will get you started on this new journey.

PART II

THE PERSONALIZED DIET PROGRAM

CHAPTER 8

Testing Your Blood Sugar Responses

Welcome to the program portion of *The Personalized Diet*. By now, you are probably very curious to learn how you react to specific foods and how you will measure that reaction. You may also be wondering whether the foods you think are good for you are actually beneficial for your blood sugar, and whether the foods you think are bad for you are maybe not so bad after all. Perhaps you are optimistic about ice cream or have your fingers crossed that broccoli should be off-limits.

As you've seen, there were plenty of surprises for the people in our study and others who have adopted the Personalized Diet. But no matter how many people's results we have seen, we cannot possibly know what your results will be. You will have to find out for yourself. It's time to investigate exactly what foods will contribute to your good health and weight management and what foods should probably be left out of your personalized healthy diet.

BLOOD SUGAR TESTING

The key to discovering your personalized diet is to test your blood sugar before and after eating the specific foods you enjoy or that you wish you could enjoy more often. Your blood sugar response is a little like a meter that registers whether many aspects of your system, including your microbiome, are reacting favorably or unfavorably to your dietary and lifestyle choices. Even without knowing what species make up your microbiome or how your genetics or health status influences your tolerance to certain foods, measuring your blood sugar can give you the broad answer: Your body will respond well to certain meals and foods with a gradual blood sugar rise and fall within a narrow range, or it will respond poorly to certain meals and foods with a dramatic blood sugar rise and fall, or it will have blood sugar that stays elevated for longer than it should. You can find out all of this information with a simple finger prick. Although a finger prick may not sound appealing, it is relatively simple and the only way for you to see in real time how your body responds to specific foods or meals.

Lucy, a colleague of ours, recently decided (at our urging) to try blood sugar testing for herself. She was hesitant about the finger pricking and what she thought would be a complicated and confusing process. She bought a blood glucose monitor "starter kit" at her local pharmacy, and once she figured out how everything worked, she tried it. She was surprised that she barely felt the prick of the tiny wire in the lancing device and at how quick and easy it was to do. Most of all, though, she was surprised at how fascinating it was to get immediate feedback on how her body responded to certain foods.

In the first week, Lucy learned that while many foods she loved, like buttered toast, red wine, and corn chips, kept her blood sugar steady, other foods, like cold cereal, pasta, and her morning mocha latte, gave her huge blood sugar spikes. Soon she was taking her testing supplies everywhere with her in her purse and testing all the foods she liked to eat regularly, as well as new foods, restaurant foods, and snack foods. She recorded detailed lists of her personal "good" and "bad" foods in her smartphone, for easy reference, and the motivation she gets from seeing those blood sugar results has been enough to keep her away from the foods that cause blood sugar spikes.

While we understand that pricking your finger may seem like a sticking point (pardon the pun), we assure you that the personalized results you will get from this experiment will be well worth the effort. You'll be glad you tried it.

It's very easy, and the more you do it, the more it seems like nothing. We have found that once people try testing their blood sugar and begin to get instant information for themselves, the more they want to learn. Some of them practice the testing for only one week, as you can do per the plan outlined in this book, but many become dedicated blood sugar testers who continually test new foods and meals and retest in different situations—such as after exercise, eating the same food at different times of day, when trying a new food or a new restaurant, or on vacation—so they can have as much information as possible about their personalized blood sugar reactions. We have seen conditions like excess weight and prediabetes resolve in many of our former study participants. If you feel unsure about using this powerful and informative health and diet tool because you will have to prick your finger, consider the following:

- The lancet is extremely thin and makes only a tiny prick in your finger. Many people say they barely feel it.
- You only have to do the blood sugar testing for one week. You can continue to test new foods if you desire, and many people find it so interesting that they continue to test as needed, but you can learn quite a bit about your personal reactions to the foods you eat over the course of only one week.
- The supplies, once costly and only for diabetics, are now quite affordable and are easily accessible without any prescription. They are available at any pharmacy, at many discount stores, and online.
- The information you will gain is invaluable and cannot be gained as precisely or accurately in any other way.
- Millions of diabetics must prick their finger many times each day to keep their blood sugar under control. Wouldn't you rather prick your finger a few times per day for one week to *avoid* diabetes?

While we think that everyone should try blood sugar testing because of the great information available from this technique, we understand that some people still may not feel they can do it. At the end of this chapter, we will talk about some other methods for evaluating your food choices, but they are more difficult, take more time, and are less precise. The gold standard for understanding how food affects you, individually, is blood sugar testing. It is the real key to understanding your personalized diet right now.

Blood Testing without the Finger Prick? Someday Soon!

In the future, there may be technology for noninvasive blood sugar measurement that will not require finger pricking, but the technology is still probably years away. There is also a company called DayTwo that licensed our personalized nutrition technology from the Weizmann Institute of Science. They have developed a method to analyze your microbiome and give you results based on a stool sample, without the need for blood sugar testing. They use this analysis to provide recommendations for meals that are most likely to be favorable to the individual, by using large databases of blood glucose responses to food, then using the algorithm we designed to predict responses. The key difference between this technology and directly testing blood sugar is that their analysis takes in several parameters, including the microbiome analysis, which together can predict reactions to foods that haven't been a part of the diet or measured by you. Also, you will get all results at once. Find out more information about how this technology works on page 305.

How to Test Your Blood Sugar

Testing your blood sugar is easy, but getting organized before you begin will make it even easier and help you avoid any unnecessary testing. In this personalized diet program, this is what you will be doing:

1. Planning what foods you want to test and shopping for what you will need.
2. Purchasing your blood sugar testing supplies.
3. Taking a practice test so you understand how to use the blood test kit.

4. Organizing your blood sugar testing schedule. You will be taking a baseline test in the mornings, then testing the foods you eat before and at intervals after eating them. (This will all be mapped out in the food testing section.)

5. Testing your blood sugar in response to specific meals and foods.

6. Tracking your results on our app, on your own, or on a chart like those provided in this book (such as on page 258).

7. Analyzing your results to determine which foods and meals work for you and which give you a blood sugar spike.

8. Enjoying your own personal "good" foods without guilt and eliminating your "bad" foods, or determining ways to modify your spike with the ideas in the next chapter.

9. Watching your weight and health measures normalize... and enjoying your life!

Let's get started!

Planning Your Test Foods

You are probably curious about how your blood sugar will respond to a number of different foods that you eat. Planning your priority test meals and foods will help you get answers in the shortest amount of time. Whether you test for one week or spread your testing out by doing fewer tests over a longer period, map out your priority test meals and foods first. We suggest testing the following:

- The meals you like to eat frequently, including all the elements you incorporate in a meal, such as a sandwich with chips and a cookie. You could test each thing separately, but if you always eat these things together, you might as well see if that combination of foods works for you. Also, if you have the same breakfast most mornings, you will want to test that.

- Individual foods you have been avoiding because you think they aren't good for you, so you can see if they might not actually be so bad for you. Test them in the serving size you would likely eat, if you knew you could eat these foods. For example, if you love ice cream or chocolate but you think you shouldn't eat them, you can test them this week to find out if they are truly bad for you.

- Individual foods (or meals) you have been eating because you think you should, although you don't enjoy them very much. If they cause a blood sugar spike, then you can happily eliminate them. If you don't particularly like oatmeal or berries or salad (and try to choke them down because they are "good" for you), test them to see if they really are as good for you as you think.

- Individual foods or beverages you are curious about, like coffee, bananas, cheese, wine, beer, or cupcakes. Eat them as snacks separately from your meals so you can test them without other foods.

- Any foods you purchase outside of the home and eat regularly. Do you have a favorite restaurant? Do you get a daily coffee order? Do you often go out for sushi, burgers, or pasta? Test those restaurant foods as well. It doesn't matter if you don't know every ingredient in the food or drink. You are not testing ingredients. Remember, this is about testing your real-life food experiences.

Meals and Foods I Want to Test

Keep track of everything you want to test here, and check off the box when you have tested it (we will show you exactly how to do the testing and record your results in the next section). This will help you keep track of everything you want to test. Note that we have included seven spaces for each meal, to fill up one week of testing. However, you don't have to test at every meal, and you can take longer than one week to test if you prefer.

Breakfast   Tested

1. _____ ☐
2. _____ ☐
3. _____ ☐
4. _____ ☐
5. _____ ☐
6. _____ ☐
7. _____ ☐

Lunch   Tested

1. _____ ☐
2. _____ ☐
3. _____ ☐
4. _____ ☐
5. _____ ☐
6. _____ ☐
7. _____ ☐

Dinner   Tested

1. _____   ☐
2. _____   ☐
3. _____   ☐
4. _____   ☐
5. _____   ☐
6. _____   ☐
7. _____   ☐

Snacks   Tested

1. _____   ☐
2. _____   ☐
3. _____   ☐
4. _____   ☐
5. _____   ☐
6. _____   ☐
7. _____   ☐

Miscellaneous Foods   Tested

1. _____   ☐
2. _____   ☐
3. _____   ☐
4. _____   ☐
5. _____   ☐
6. _____   ☐
7. _____   ☐

Purchasing Your Supplies

Before you can begin testing your blood sugar, you will need some supplies. Because people with diabetes need to monitor their blood sugar, blood sugar testing supplies have been available over the counter for many years, but these supplies were traditionally expensive (and were covered by insurance). However, blood testing supplies have become much more affordable in recent years, not just because more people have diabetes than ever before but probably also because blood sugar testing has become more popular with biohackers (people who like to experiment with what affects their health), low-carb dieters, and others who want to know what their blood sugar does. Also, blood sugar testing has gone high-tech, making it easier and more accessible to everyone, with Bluetooth or wired blood glucose meters and associated apps for mobile phones and computers.

Everything you will need can probably be found together in one kit, for between $20 and $50. Search "blood sugar testing supplies" online, or shop around at local pharmacies or discount stores for the best deal. There are many options, and the costs will probably continue to go down as blood sugar testing continues to get more popular. Here are all the components you need:

- **Blood glucose meter.** These can be quite simple and inexpensive, or higher tech. Some even synchronize to your smartphone via Bluetooth and automatically track your test results.
- **Lancing device and lancets.** These are simple and inexpensive. You need only one lancing device, and large packs of lancets last a long time.

- **Blood glucose test strips.** This is the most expensive item, and because strips are specific to the blood glucose meter, it's best to find a good deal on the strips first and then buy a glucose meter to match. Over-the-counter test strips are all nearly equal in terms of accuracy, so it's okay to shop according to price, which can vary widely. A bottle of 100 strips could cost up to $200 from a pharmacy, but you can also find boxes of 50 strips for as little as $10 or $12. At five to six measurements per meal, that's just about $1 per meal in testing expense.

Taking a Practice Test

Once you have your supplies, you will be ready to start testing. Before you launch into your food testing, try the test once or twice so you understand how to use the equipment. It may seem complex at first, but once you do it, you will see how easy it is. Follow the directions for the supplies you purchased—each has its own procedure—but in general, this is what you will be doing:

1. Turn on the monitor. (If applicable, also turn on the app on your phone, if it synchronizes with your monitor.)
2. When prompted, put a test strip into the monitor.
3. Load a lancet into the lancing device.
4. Put your finger against the lancing device and press the button to lightly prick your finger.
5. Touch your finger to the end of the test strip. You need only a tiny drop of blood.
6. Wait for the monitor to register your blood sugar reading. This typically takes only a few seconds.

7. Record the results, along with the time and situation (e.g., first thing in the morning, 30 minutes after XX food, and so on).

When you first begin testing, we recommend a calibration phase. Test your blood sugar two to three times in a row to see if you get similar results—they should be within 10 to 20 mg/dL or (for diabetics) at higher levels in the 10 to 20 mg/dL range; the results should be within 10 to 20 percent of each other. Such deviations are normal because there are many influences on your results—how you did the pricking, the size of the blood drop, even air temperature. These are all just "measurement noise," and of no concern if your results range within the above parameters. Home blood sugar tests are not quite as precise as those that doctors use, and this much variation is normal. If you get a large variation once, that's probably just an error, but if you do multiple tests in a row and they continue to be all over the place (greater than 20 percent apart), the meter may be faulty and you should exchange it for a new one.

Once you start testing, you can consider rises beyond 10 to 20 percent of your level prior to eating to be valid signals coming from the food you ate. This will allow you to take good measurements. If you find that you occasionally get an extremely high or extremely low measurement, this could also be an error. Try taking the measurement again (see page 266 for more about what to do when this happens).

Once you get in the habit of testing your own blood sugar, you will find it is quick and easy to do. If you carry your supplies in a pouch with you, you can test anywhere and anytime, as necessary.

Organizing Your Testing Schedule

There are many ways to organize your testing schedule, depending on how often you want to test. You could test every meal and snack for a week, or test just one meal every day for several weeks, until you've tested everything you want to test. Or, you could do something in between.

The first thing to work into your schedule is establishing your fasting blood sugar. This measures your blood sugar first thing in the morning, before you eat anything, and it will serve as a baseline so you can see how different foods affect your blood sugar from that baseline. This is very important because every time you test a meal, you will be tracking the rise and fall of your blood sugar. If you know your baseline, you will know when your blood sugar is back to normal. How long it takes for your blood sugar to return to normal is as important in your blood sugar testing as how high your blood sugar goes after consuming a particular food.

When you have decided to test a particular meal or snack, you will need to test your blood sugar once right before eating. If it is not at or close to your fasting blood sugar level (the number you got when you tested first thing in the morning), then you wait to test until it has gone back to normal. Sometimes your level can be too high if you ate something recently. You should always start a test at or near your baseline.

Then you will be doing four separate tests after eating, in 30-minute increments, starting 30 minutes after your first bite of food. In other words, you will be testing at 30, 60, 90, and 120 minutes. If your blood sugar is still elevated after 2 hours, continue testing every 30 minutes until it is within 10 to 20 percent of your fasting blood sugar reading from first thing in the morning.

For example, your baseline, fasting blood sugar is 85 mg/dL. (It won't be exactly the same every morning, but it should be close.) Assuming you eat breakfast soon after getting up, your fasting blood sugar can count as your before-breakfast reading. After your first bite of breakfast, start timing. At 30 minutes, take another measure. Your blood sugar might be at 120 mg/dL. At 60 minutes, it might be at 100 mg/dL. At 90 minutes, it might be at 95 mg/dL. At 2 hours, it should be back to approximately 85 mg/dL.

Your individual readings might be quite different from this example. Yours might go up much higher. It might come back down to baseline by 60 minutes. It might not go up very high but might stay elevated for longer. These fluctuations can happen for many reasons, including your own health parameters, microbiome composition, time of day, and, of course, the foods you eat. But what really matters is how *you* respond to that breakfast *you* like to eat.

At first, you won't know if your blood sugar is spiking because this is individual to you. If your blood sugar *always* goes up to approximately 120 mg/dL after eating, then this is typical for you. But if a food suddenly takes you up to 160 mg/dL, then that would be a spike. If you are diabetic, your typical rise may be higher—for instance, if your typical rise is 160/dL, then a post-meal glucose response that suddenly went over 200 mg/dL would be considered a spike for you. The more you test, the more you will get a sense of what is normal for you and what isn't. (This will be easy to track and discern using our free app.)

Are Your Results "Normal"?

It is one thing for us to tell you to learn what is normal *for you*, but you are probably wondering how you will know whether your blood sugar levels are normal *in general*, or if they indicate the

possibility that you might be prediabetic or diabetic. This is important. Some people in our study found out they were prediabetic
or diabetic because they were testing their blood sugar.

While occasional blood sugar spikes happen to everyone
and can be food- and situation-specific, if your blood sugar is
consistently above a certain level, then that can warrant a visit
to your doctor for further testing. According to the American
Diabetes Association, these are the fasting and postmeal blood
sugar guidelines:

Fasting Blood Sugar Numbers	
Normal, for a person without diabetes	70–99 mg/dL
Prediabetic range	100–125 mg/dL
Diabetic range	Above 125 mg/dL
ADA recommended goal for diabetics	80–130 mg/dL

Blood Sugar Numbers 2 Hours after Meal	
Normal, for a person without diabetes	Less than 140 mg/dL
Prediabetic range	140–199 mg/dL
Diabetic range	Above 200 mg/dL
ADA recommended goal for diabetics	Less than 180 mg/dL

Remember that while the overall goal is to get your blood
sugar into the normal range, the point of testing individual meals
and foods is to determine which foods give you the healthiest
response. Choosing those foods will help to nudge your blood
sugar spikes downward. This will likely bring your fasting levels
down eventually, too.

Ideal Testing Schedule

This is the schedule we recommend:

- Upon waking (to establish a baseline)
- 30 minutes after the first bite of breakfast
- 60 minutes after breakfast
- 90 minutes after breakfast
- 120 minutes after breakfast
- Before lunch
- 30 minutes after the first bite of lunch
- 60 minutes after lunch
- 90 minutes after lunch
- 120 minutes after lunch
- Before afternoon snack (if you have one)
- 30 minutes after the first bite of snack
- 60 minutes after snack
- 90 minutes after snack
- 120 minutes after snack
- Before dinner
- 30 minutes after the first bite of dinner
- 60 minutes after dinner
- 90 minutes after dinner
- 120 minutes after dinner
- Before and after any other snacks, as you would for a meal, including late-night snacks
- Right before going to bed, to see if you have gotten back to baseline

This may sound like a lot of testing, but the more you test, the more information you will have. Again, remember you don't have to test every meal and snack every day. If you want to spread your testing out over a longer period, that is just as effective.

The Importance of Getting Back to Baseline

To get the most accurate assessment of a meal or food from blood sugar testing, your blood sugar should be at baseline *before* you eat. Baseline is within 10 to 20 mg/dL of your standard fasting or waking blood sugar reading that you will take first thing in the morning. If you test prior to a meal and your blood sugar is higher than this (which can happen especially if you are eating meals too close together), your blood sugar result won't necessarily be reliable. If your before-meal reading is more than 10 to 20 mg/dL of your baseline, we recommend either not bothering to test that meal or waiting to eat it until your blood sugar has returned to baseline.

Because how and when you eat may be different from other people, you can also adjust your testing schedule to suit your needs or the demands on your time. Here are two other options:

Testing Schedule Option #1

If you do not want to test every meal or snack, but instead would rather test only certain meals or snacks throughout the day, and eat without testing the rest of the time, you can follow this option. Maybe you will test only one day a week or maybe just a few days per week. If that's your preference, follow this schedule, which you can do for several weeks, or you can do this randomly for as long as it is productive for you:

- Upon waking (to establish a baseline)
- Just before any meal or food you want to test

- 30 minutes after the first bite of that meal or food
- 60 minutes after
- 90 minutes after
- 120 minutes after
- Right before going to bed, to see if you have returned to baseline

TESTING SCHEDULE OPTION #2

Another option is to test all your meals but not to do as many tests before or after those meals. This testing approach won't give you as much information about the rise and fall of your blood sugar, but it will give you good basic information so you will know where the real issues are. If that's your preference, try this schedule:

- Upon waking (to establish a baseline)
- Right before eating a meal or snack
- 60 minutes after the first bite of any meal or food
- 120 minutes after

Whatever testing schedule you choose, have a plan and know that it will give you more information than you had before.

Start Testing and Tracking Your Results

Now that you have everything ready, it's time to start testing according to your food plan and testing schedule. As you go, you will be tracking your results so you can analyze them. There are two ways to do this: through our app, which you can download from our website at www.thepersonalizeddiet.com, or on your own. Of course, we highly recommend using our app because it is a much easier way to keep track of your data. It stores everything and will compute your responses from the raw data you enter. It will summarize your responses to meals and provide other summaries of your nutritional intake. And it's free! It can work on any smartphone. Again, you can download it at www.thepersonalizeddiet.com. You're going to like using it because:

- The app keeps all the data and information organized for you. You will select the food components of the meal you are eating from a database of more than 10,000 foods. This database includes nutritional values (calories, carbs, fat, protein, vitamins, and minerals), which is an added bonus because it will help you to ascertain whether your meals are balanced and that you are not overeating on a regular basis. The app can also calculate your personal caloric and nutritional needs.

- The app will remind you when to test.

- The app will take the blood sugar measurements you enter and show you a graph of your blood sugar response, along with a score for each meal that takes into account the length of the rise as well as the height of the rise. This scoring system makes it easy to see which meals were favorable and which were unfavorable.

- The app will keep all the meals organized for you, creating a list of all the meals that you have tested, along with the score provided for each meal. You will be able to sort that list and see it anytime you want, so you can easily recall which foods and meals were "good" and which were "bad."

We think this app will be extremely useful and will take a lot of the work out of keeping your information logged and organized.

However, if you prefer to create your own system, that is fine. Keep track of all your results and record when you did the tests. You could do this in a chart and then log the numbers into a graph, by hand or in a graphing program like PowerPoint. This will give you a record of what you ate and when, and will provide a visual representation of which lines are about normal for you and which ones go up much higher or stay up much longer than usual. These higher/longer rises are your blood sugar spikes and indicate your "bad" foods or meals.

Here is an example of some of the ways you might track this information on your own, if you really don't want to use the app.

SAMPLE HOMEMADE BLOOD SUGAR TRACKING CHART

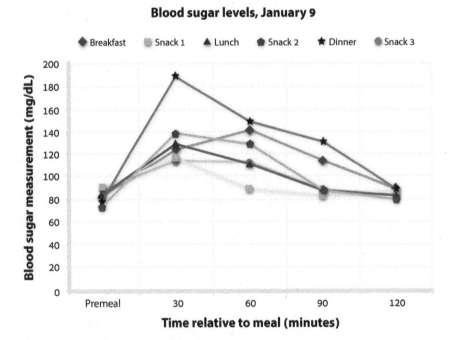

Breakfast:	Snack 1:	Lunch:	Snack 2:	Dinner:	Snack 3:
Oatmeal with berries, coffee with cream	Apple with almond butter	Turkey sand-wich, potato chips	Orange	Lentil curry, basmati rice, samosa, yogurt drink	Chocolate ice cream

If you like numbers more than graphics, you could also make a table like what is below, where you can list your numbers.

	Breakfast: Oatmeal with berries, coffee with cream	Snack 1: Apple with almond butter	Lunch: Turkey sandwich, potato chips	Snack 2: Orange	Dinner: Lentil curry, basmati rice, samosa, yogurt drink	Snack 3: Chocolate ice cream
Premeal	84	91	84	75	79	90
30 min	125	118	130	140	190	115
60 min	142	90	112	130	150	114
90 min	115	84	90	89	132	90
120 min	90	88	85	80	90	84

However, we created the app to take the burden off you for creating your own charts or system. We hope you will use it!

Organizing Your Data

After you have tracked your reactions to all the different meals and foods on your list on page 244, it's time to look at your list of good meals and foods (the ones that resulted in only a gentle rise in blood sugar) and your bad meals and foods (the ones that resulted in a more dramatic spike in blood sugar). If you have been using the app, this has all been done for you and you have scores that show you which foods are good and bad for you. If you have been tracking your data on your own, you could organize that information for yourself like this:

Tested Meal/Food	Bad or Good?

Breakfast:

1. _____   _____
2. _____   _____
3. _____   _____
4. _____   _____
5. _____   _____
6. _____   _____
7. _____   _____

Lunch:

1. _____   _____
2. _____   _____
3. _____   _____
4. _____   _____
5. _____   _____
6. _____   _____
7. _____   _____

Dinner:

1. _____   _____
2. _____   _____
3. _____   _____

4. _____   _____
5. _____   _____
6. _____   _____
7. _____   _____

Snacks:

1. _____   _____
2. _____   _____
3. _____   _____
4. _____   _____
5. _____   _____
6. _____   _____
7. _____   _____

Miscellaneous/Individual Foods:

1. _____   _____
2. _____   _____
3. _____   _____
4. _____   _____
5. _____   _____
6. _____   _____
7. _____   _____

Nadav G.

I feel lucky to have heard about the Personalized Nutrition Project at the Weizmann Institute because I took part in the study and it changed my life. When I changed my eating habits to feature the foods that were good for me (like apples, quinoa, hummus, most soup, sushi, and chocolate!) and eliminated the foods that were bad for me (including cereal, bananas, pasta, and doughnuts), I lost 18 pounds! I don't miss the foods that are bad for me because seeing my blood sugar reaction made me lose my taste for them, knowing what they were doing to me. I've been implementing the changes for more than a year now and haven't gained any weight back.

IF YOU CAN'T OR WON'T TEST YOUR BLOOD SUGAR

If you want to get your blood sugar under control, but you really don't want to test your own blood sugar, or cannot do so for some reason, there is another way you can get a fairly good, if less precise, idea of how specific meals and foods affect your blood sugar. That is to track your hunger levels and weight. In general, hunger after eating, when you should be satiated, is a sign of blood sugar going too high and then dropping too low due to an insulin surge.[1,2] In other words, a blood sugar spike. In general, weight gain is a sign that your blood sugar has been going too high, causing insulin to surge and causing more fat storage. Hunger, as you can see, is a more immediate indication of blood sugar, while weight gain is a longer-term indication that your diet in general is contributing to fat storage—likely through the mechanism of excess insulin production in response to high blood sugar.

To track your hunger, you can keep track of how hungry you are at intervals after each meal or snack. We like to use the following numerical scale:

1. Not hungry at all
2. Mildly hungry
3. Moderately hungry
4. Very hungry
5. Extremely hungry

Record your hunger before you eat, and 1, 2, and 3 hours after you eat. The app can also do this for you—it includes a hunger tracking function. Then you can organize the results on the app (download it at www.thepersonalizeddiet.com), or you can do it on your own by making your own chart or table, which could look something like this:

	Hunger level before	Hunger level 1 hour after	Hunger level 2 hours after	Hunger level 3 hours after
Breakfast				
Snack				
Lunch				
Snack				
Dinner				
Snack				

You can also graph these falls and rises in the same way you do for blood sugar numbers, although this graph will be simpler. Or you can just look at the numbers: Foods that result in hunger after eating them correlate loosely to higher blood sugar spikes. The higher the number and/or the longer the number stays high (the longer you stay hungry), the higher the spike. Foods that do not make you feel hungry after eating them correlate to low blood sugar rises. This can help you determine which foods are best for you and which foods may be causing harm.

Another even less precise but possibly effective way to track your blood sugar is through weight gain and loss. For this method, keep track of what you eat every day. Then, once every week, record your weight. It will take more than one week to get an indication of what's going on because weight responds more slowly. Also, because weight responds to so many different factors, it can be difficult to tell what is causing any weight gain. However, in general you can try different foods or combinations of foods and see if your weight responds positively or negatively.

Again, the app can keep track of this for you, along with how many calories you have been eating between weekly weight recordings if you want to know that, although we don't encourage focusing too much on calories, other than as a general indication that you aren't overeating. You should be more interested in which foods affect your blood sugar, rather than how many calories you are taking in. However, some people like to keep track of this.

You can track your weight yourself, but again, this will be much less precise. If you have been eating many carbs and gaining weight, you could try cutting back. Or you could try different carbs, or eating more fiber, or consuming more or less fat. Without blood sugar testing, your experiments will be much more general and less informative.

If you don't test your blood sugar, we suggest using the hunger and weight methods together. Do what works best for you, and know that you can still use the app.

FREQUENTLY ASKED QUESTIONS ABOUT BLOOD SUGAR TESTING

The following are some questions we have been asked about blood testing. You may have similar questions before you start testing and once you are testing regularly, whether it is for the one week or if you choose to extend your testing time.

1. ***Does the finger prick hurt?***

   Barely at all, although it depends on your sensitivity. Many people say they hardly feel the finger stick. Others are more sensitive to it, but do it anyway because the information they get is worthwhile. We have very rarely encountered someone who stops testing due to discomfort.

2. ***What is a normal blood sugar level before eating and at 30, 60, 90, and 120 minutes?***

   The American Diabetes Association only specifies what fasting blood sugar numbers and blood sugar numbers should be 2 hours after meals (see page 251). You can find many different opinions about what numbers should be at other times, from 15 minutes after eating to 3 hours after eating. However, there is not an official consensus on this. We advise you not to worry about how your measures stack up against one number for each test. Instead, look at the whole arc of your blood sugar rise. If it goes up extremely high compared to other numbers, consider that a spike. If it goes up and stays up for a long time before coming back down to normal compared to other numbers, that may also be a sign that the meal or food is not a good one for you.

3. *I've noticed that my blood sugar rises, falls, and then rises again after a meal. Shouldn't it just go up and then down?*

Your pancreas releases insulin in two stages. When it first senses a rise in blood sugar from food, your beta cells kick in and begin releasing insulin. This is called a *first-phase insulin release*. Sometimes the amount of insulin is enough to process the blood sugar from your meal. If it isn't enough—maybe you ate a big meal or continued eating for a long time—then your pancreas will typically release more insulin, called a *second-phase insulin release*. This should be enough to get your blood sugar back down to your baseline level before your next meal.

4. *What if my meal lasts for more than 30 minutes, has multiple courses, or ends with dessert? Do I still start counting my 30 minutes from the beginning of the meal and test before it's over?*

If your meal will last longer than 30 minutes, you should start measuring as soon as you start the meal and then measure every 30 minutes (even if you aren't done eating yet, if possible), until 90 minutes after ending the meal. You can then examine the glucose graph across this entire period. These analyses are highly useful and will tell you how you respond to a longer meal. However, this approach may be less helpful in determining what part of the meal caused any spikes. The more food or courses you eat, the more factors are at play.

5. *Sometimes I have dessert, but I don't want it immediately after dinner. What happens if I eat dessert 30 to 60 minutes after a dinner? How does that affect testing?*

    If the dessert is 60 minutes after the start of the meal, then you can still test and evaluate the first 90 minutes after the start of dinner, because the effect of the dessert will take around 30 minutes to kick in. If the dessert is within 30 minutes, then you can consider it part of the dinner and this would be like testing the response to a more complex meal (see previous question). You should then measure until 90 minutes after the dessert. If the dessert is more than an hour after your meal, you can measure it separately, as an individual item—although if your blood sugar is not back to your baseline before eating dessert, the measurement may not be as accurate as it would be if you ate it alone.

6. *What if I eat again before my blood sugar is back to normal, or within 2 hours of another meal? How do I time my testing?*

    In this case, you can still measure the meal, but you should consider that your response is not the response you would expect to see if you ate it when your blood sugar was back to baseline. Rather, you should treat it as the response that you would get if you ate this meal after the previous meal you just ate. This is useful to show you what happens if you eat meals close together. If frequent eating tends to spike your blood sugar, then you know that it is better to wait until your blood sugar is back to baseline to eat again.

7. *I had a very high blood sugar spike after 30 minutes, but my blood sugar was back down to normal by 1 hour. Is that something to worry about?*

Sometimes you may get a reading that seems unusually high (such as over 200 mg/dL) or unusually low (such as below 60 mg/dL). If these readings are accurate and happen often, you should consult with your family physician about the results. However, extreme readings recorded once that don't repeat themselves are often not real. Testing kits can also make errors for any number of reasons. There may not have been quite enough blood on the sample, the sample was mixed with something, or there was a meter malfunction. Let's say you ate a cupcake and had a little sugar on your hand when you handled the test strip. That alone could skew your results dramatically and inaccurately. If you get a reading that seems much too low or much too high, take another one. If the second reading is much closer to normal, assume that reading is the correct one. If the reading remains very high or very low after three tests, it is probably accurate. However, even then, it isn't clear that occasional low or high numbers are critical or matter that much. Generally, we look at the total rise over time of blood sugar after a meal, and that is the basis of the score we give on the app. A quick rise that falls back down to normal quickly wouldn't register as particularly significant. What's most important is how you compare to yourself across different meals over time. Does your blood sugar often act this way, or is it unusual for you? However, if you are frequently getting extremely high or low numbers with several tests, then give your doctor a call (see the next question).

8. *At what point should I talk to my doctor, if I think my fasting (waking) blood sugar or postmeal blood sugar results are too high?*

If your fasting (waking) or postmeal blood sugar results are consistently in the prediabetic or diabetic range as indicated in the charts on page 251, then it is a good idea to talk to your doctor, who can give you a fasting blood sugar test, and possibly a glucose response test, to determine if you have a medical issue. Because you are taking periodic measurements, you have more information than a doctor who is taking only a snapshot (based on one test in the office), so if you have been seeing consistently high numbers, that is useful information for your doctor. And a diagnosis is important, if you are prediabetic or diabetic, so you can respond appropriately to bring your blood sugar back down. You can often do this with diet, but in some cases, you might require medication. There are many options for treating these conditions, which don't all involve taking insulin, but only your doctor can help you decide what treatment is appropriate for you.

9. *Can I tell the state of my blood sugar just by how I feel?*

While you may have read that both high blood sugar and low blood sugar are often accompanied by certain sensations or feelings, like dizziness, shakiness, fatigue, or brain fog, in our experience, these feelings are too vague to be reliable. In fact, people have told us that they sometimes feel dizzy or shaky or tired and are sure their blood sugar is going to be very low (such as below 70 mg/dL, the upper limit for hypoglycemia) or very high (such as over 200 mg/dL after a meal), only to discover it is completely within a normal range. There are many reasons people feel dizzy, shaky, fatigued, or foggy that may have nothing to do with blood sugar. It's better to test and know for sure.

If you consistently notice certain symptoms associated with low or high blood sugar and you verify that your blood sugar is low or high when you feel that way, you may be able to rely on those feelings in the future. This is just one more aspect of getting to understand and tune in to your own reactions to food. If you have been recording the foods you are eating, you can also objectively document if these higher or lower levels and associated "symptoms" occur consistently after certain meals. You will have the opportunity to log these kinds of responses in the app, or you can keep track of them on your own.

10. *If I keep my blood sugar under control, can I eat as much as I want and lose weight?*

Of course not. If you take in a lot more energy than your body needs, regardless of blood sugar, you will store that extra energy as fat. If you do this regularly, you will eventually start gaining weight. Although we explained why not all calories are the same (see page 109), it is important to remember that while eating meals that cause lower blood sugar rises is better for avoiding weight gain and aiding in weight loss, that doesn't mean the amount of energy in the food you eat (i.e., calories) is not important at all. For one thing, excessive food intake is more likely to cause a blood sugar spike. You may discover that if you eat a moderate portion of a food you like, you will not get a blood sugar spike, but if you eat a very large portion of that same food, you may get a blood sugar spike. Portion size affects blood sugar rise, and we saw a correlation in our study between calorie content and postmeal blood sugar response. But even if a large amount of a certain food does not result in a blood sugar spike for you, it can still result in you taking in too much energy. Keeping a balanced diet in terms of vitamins and minerals and eating moderate portions according to your energy needs instead of overeating well beyond your energy needs will also help with health and avoiding weight gain. Again, we don't want you to overfocus on calories, and this is always a temptation since dieters have been conditioned to count calories. However, we want you to pay more attention to the specific foods that are causing you a problem. This will be easier to do if your calorie intake is moderate. Keeping your blood sugar rises low and cutting back even a little bit on portions that maintain your weight may even help you to lose weight easily.

11. I've seen HbA1c tests in the pharmacy with the blood sugar testing supplies. Should I do this test, too?

The HbA1c test is one of the primary tests for diagnosing diabetes. It shows your general blood sugar control over the previous two months before the test. You may choose to perform an HbA1c home test if you are worried that you might have prediabetes or diabetes. Traditionally, this is a test your doctor would do, although it may not be covered by your insurance if you don't have any symptoms (such as high fasting blood sugar) to warrant the test. If you don't have a medical reason to have the test, you can buy it in a pharmacy and check it out for yourself. Like the blood sugar test, it requires finger pricking, but just once, and the test only needs to be repeated around every three to six months. It costs about $40.

If you decide you want to try it, an HbA1c level below 5.7 percent is considered normal. HbA1c of 5.7 to 6.5 percent is considered within the prediabetic range, while HbA1c of over 6.5 percent is considered a diabetic reading. If you get an abnormal reading, this is something to ask your doctor about. In such a case, your physician will likely repeat the test to ensure that it is accurate and correct—no single blood test is flawless. Also, remember that no matter where you are—normal, prediabetic, or diabetic—it is always beneficial to your health to choose foods that don't spike your blood sugar levels relative to the other foods you eat.

By the way, the HbA1c test is in no way informative regarding the effects of specific foods. It is an average of your blood glucose levels over the past two months or so. A high HbA1c may mean you tend to respond with higher blood sugar levels to food in general, but it is always best to know what foods spike you, so you can make the best choices for your diet. Over time, keeping your blood sugar more level is likely to help you lower an elevated HbA1c.

If you have no reason to suspect, based on your blood sugar testing numbers, that you might have prediabetes or diabetes, we certainly wouldn't worry about this test, as it is somewhat expensive compared to blood sugar testing.

12. *Why did my blood sugar spike after eating a food at one meal, and then not when I ate the same food at another meal?*

There are many factors that can alter your responses, including the time of day, whether you exercised before or after eating the food, what you ate or drank along with the food, even the time of your hormonal cycle. For example, pasta with salad and a glass of wine may result in a much different result than pasta with garlic bread or a second helping of pasta. For this reason, it is helpful to test spiking foods in various situations. We will talk more about this in the next few chapters.

CHAPTER 9

Fine-Tuning Your Personalized Diet

Amy loves toast. She loves it with eggs, she loves it with jam, she loves it with peanut butter, and most of all, she loves it with cultured French butter. For Amy, two slices of sourdough toast with French butter and a hot cup of coffee with cream is breakfast heaven. However, Amy believed that she should be eating less fat, so to lose some weight, she often skipped toast in favor of grapefruit and oatmeal, ate the toast with tomatoes and cucumber slices, or had toast dry. It wasn't what she wanted, but it was what she thought she should do.

After testing her blood sugar, Amy discovered that oatmeal and grapefruit gave her a very large blood sugar spike in the morning. She was secretly relieved, because she never liked that breakfast very much anyway. And when she tried testing her toast, in its plain dry state, it also gave her a spike—not as large as the oatmeal and grapefruit, but still larger than she liked to see. Then she decided to see what would happen if she spread cultured French butter on her toast. She made two slices of her favorite sourdough toast and slathered it with a generous amount of French butter. And as long as she was throwing caution to the wind, she decided to put the cream she loved so much back into the coffee she had been drinking black. She enjoyed every bite, every sip...and then was overjoyed to discover that her favorite breakfast—toast with butter and coffee with cream—didn't spike her blood sugar. Not after 30 minutes. Not after 60 minutes. Not at all.

We suspect this is because fat tends to blunt blood sugar spikes, a phenomenon we noticed in our study. It doesn't do this for everyone, but for many people, fat is a blood sugar ally and just one of many ways you can manipulate your own blood sugar spikes to bring them down and possibly be able to enjoy your favorite foods, even if they spiked your blood sugar when you tested them. Sometimes, eating a food the way you like it (and not the way you *think* it should be eaten for weight loss or health) results in a more favorable blood sugar response. This is not always the case, but sometimes it happens—and wouldn't you like to know if that is the case for you?

Once you've finished your week of testing, you have some valuable information. You know which meals and foods make your blood sugar go too high, and you know which meals and foods cause only a gentle rise or no rise at all. You may also still want to test new meals and foods you discover from time to time, and that's fantastic. Many of the people in our study have gone on to test new foods, so they can continue to tweak and adjust their diets in a way that works specifically for them.

You know your good foods and your bad foods...but what if the idea of giving up some of your bad foods is too painful? Would you like to find a way to eat that food you love, despite it spiking your blood sugar when you tested it?

From our study, we observed many trends about things that made blood sugar *tend* to go higher or lower, including particular types of carbs, added fat, added fiber, salt, water, exercise, sleep, and so on. Using what we discovered, you can try out these strategies out to see if you can get your spikes to come down. In some cases, the food itself may not have been the primary cause of the spike. It might have been that you didn't get enough sleep, or added too much salt, or perhaps the spike would come down if you changed the type of carb or added fat. Let's look at all those options and see how we can hack your blood sugar spikes. If they stay high no matter what you try, then that meal or food really may not be right for you. If, however, you can get your blood sugar to come down, then you can add them back into your dietary rotation with an easy conscience.

You kept track of everything you tried on the chart on page 258 so you could determine what foods were and were not good for you, personally. Now look back at the foods that caused spikes. You may be able to modify those spikes and work those foods back into your diet.

Let's look at how, starting with carbohydrate manipulation.

CARBOHYDRATES

To put it simply, carbohydrates are molecules made of carbon ("carb"), oxygen ("o"), and hydrogen ("hydrate"). There are many kinds of carbohydrates—monosaccharides, disaccharides, oligosaccharides, polysaccharides—but essentially, and for nutritional purposes, they are starches, sugars, and fiber. Foods that have a high proportion of starch, sugar, and/or fiber are considered carbohydrate-rich foods, which many people shorten to "carbs," as in, "I'm trying to limit my carbs," or "Oh, how I love carbs!"

Carbohydrates are also considered, in nutrition science, to be one of three macronutrients, or primary nutrients in food. The other two macronutrients are protein and fat. Carbohydrates provide quick as well as stored energy. There are also certain types of carbohydrates that your body doesn't digest, such as fiber and other polysaccharides. They go directly to the gut bacteria, where they influence the success or failure of various microbiome species (they also do other things like facilitate the elimination of waste products). People who eat so-called high-carb diets tend to have different microbiome profiles than people who eat low-carb diets. For example, diets containing a lot of sugar (monosaccharides and disaccharides), or sugar and fat, tend to promote gut bacteria that may have certain adverse health effects, such as increased fat storage[1] or decreased cognitive flexibility.[2] Diets containing fiber-rich complex carbohydrates (oligosaccharides and polysaccharides) tend to have more microbiome diversity[3] and may be related to better health status, such as reducing obesity and decreasing inflammation.[4,5,6] Keep in mind that these are only tendencies and, while interesting, are not always true. The microbiome is complex and influenced by many factors. We don't yet know everything about what shapes it and changes it. This is an active area of research, but it is interesting to note the effect carbohydrates may sometimes have on the microbiome.

You may have already discovered from your blood sugar testing that some carbohydrate-rich foods tend to give you a blood sugar spike and others don't. For example, in our study, we found that one person experienced a blood sugar spike from cookies but not from bananas, while another person experienced a blood sugar spike from bananas but not from cookies (see page 225). As an example, let's say you spike when you eat bananas, but you *love* bananas. Or, maybe you spike when you eat rice, but you love rice and can't imagine life without it. What if toast or oatmeal gives you a spike, but you don't want to switch to eating eggs every morning? Or maybe it's that evening cocktail that sends your blood sugar skyrocketing. Do you have to become a teetotaler?

The good news is you don't have to abandon the food you love altogether. Restrictive diets that prohibit you from eating favorite foods often don't work because they are too difficult to follow over the long term. But what do you do if you want to enjoy a carbohydrate-containing meal that tends to spike your blood sugar? One good way is to test the same meal with a different carbohydrate. We call this *carb swapping*, and here are some ways to do it. Take the meal or food you want to be able to eat, and do the following:

- **Isolate the offender.** If the spiking meal contains multiple carbs, the first thing you could do is test it several times, eliminating one of the carbs each time you test, so you can figure out which carb (or carbs) is the offender. (Our app contains nutritional values for all the foods, so if you aren't sure if a food is carb-heavy or not, you can find that information there.) For example, let's say you want to eat oatmeal in the morning, and you usually have it with milk and sugar, with a side of orange juice. Which carb is causing you the problem? Is it the oatmeal, the milk, the sugar, or the orange juice? You could try the oatmeal with milk but no toppings. Then you could try orange juice alone. Then you could try oatmeal with raisins instead of sugar. For each option, test your blood sugar at 30, 60, 90, and 120 minutes (or assess your hunger level after eating it). This can help you zoom in on the glucose-spiking ingredients. Then you know which thing to eliminate or swap. You could keep track of these experiments in a chart like this:

MEAL	30 min	60 min	90 min	120 min
Oatmeal, skim milk, sugar, orange juice				
Oatmeal, soy milk, raisins				
Orange juice only				
Oatmeal, no milk, fresh fruit				

- **Reduce the portion.** If you love to eat a big bowl of oatmeal (or pasta or rice or whatever grain you like), would you be happy with a small bowl? If not, then don't bother with this test, but if you think you would be just as happy with less, try adjusting your serving size. It may be the amount that is causing the spike, rather than the actual food items. You could track this experiment like this:

MEAL	30 min	60 min	90 min	120 min
2 cups spaghetti with meat sauce				
1 cup spaghetti with meat sauce				
½ cup spaghetti with meat sauce				

- **Break up the meal.** If you increase the duration of your meal, you may decrease your blood sugar rise. You could try eating more slowly or breaking a large meal into portions or courses and waiting a short while between courses (this is what dinner conversation is for). Or you could eat more frequent, smaller meals throughout the day instead of fewer, larger meals (this also takes advantage of the blood-sugar-lowering properties of smaller meals).
- **Manipulate your grain.** If the oats are the problem (or the rice or the wheat or whatever grain you are eating in the problematic meal), try substituting a different type of grain or substituting half or all your grains for legumes (legumes tend to have lower glucose rises in general). There are many kinds of grains and legumes, so break out of your rut and try some new types. Some people are very carb-sensitive and don't do well with any grain, but

more often we find that there are some grains that work for most people. If the first grain swap doesn't work, try another one, such as the following:

Amaranth

Barley

Brown rice: short grain, basmati, long grain

Buckwheat

Cornmeal/polenta

Millet

Oats: old-fashioned, Irish, steel-cut

Quinoa

Rye

Sorghum

Spelt

Teff

Triticale

Wheat berries

White rice: short grain, basmati, jasmine, long grain

Adzuki beans

Black beans

Black-eyed peas

Butter beans

Cannellini beans

Chickpeas / garbanzo beans

Green peas

Kidney beans

Lentils: brown, red, green

Lima beans

Navy beans

Peanuts / peanut butter

Pinto beans

Soybeans

Ran B.

I am an avid marathon runner and I spend many hours training. Like my friend Eran Segal, I have always been interested in how nutrition could enhance my athletic performance, as well as my postexercise recovery. There are a lot of clichés, myths, tips, secrets, and recipes floating around in the world of runners, and sometimes it's difficult to know what to believe. We all know we need to eat food for energy, but we also don't want to have to carry any extra weight with us as we run a marathon, compete in a triathlon, or whatever the event might be.

I've often experimented with different types of diets to see how they would influence me. I had heard that some people, including Eran, had a very good result with a low-carb diet, but for me, reducing my carbohydrate intake drastically had an immediate negative effect. I felt weaker during training. However, I decided to try diversifying the carbs I was eating. I often have to eat away from home, and rice was my carb of choice on most days. When I experimented with replacing rice with quinoa, I noticed an almost immediate result. I had more energy, my performance was just as good, and without reducing my calories, I lost almost 5 pounds. Now I feel leaner, stronger, and more energetic, just from swapping one carb for another.

- **Increase fiber.** In our study, we saw that in many cases, although adding fiber to a meal tended to raise the immediate postmeal blood sugar response, it also tended to lower the postmeal blood sugar response of a meal the following day. Try including more fiber to your meal, such as using whole grains instead of refined grains, or adding wheat bran, oat bran, wheat germ, or another fiber-rich addition to a fruit smoothie or yogurt, for example. Do this for several days in a row, and then retest the meal.
- **Manipulate your fruit.** If you discover or suspect that fruit is the problem, try a different fruit. Dried fruits contain concentrated sugars, so you may find that substituting fresh fruit (such as adding blueberries to your oatmeal instead of raisins) makes a difference. If you enjoy fruit for your snacks but bananas spike you, try apples. If

oranges spike you, try mangoes. It's always beneficial to add more diversity to your diet, and trying more fruits will also give you the added benefit of additional nutrients. In general, berries tend to have the lowest amount of sugar. You may find they are the fruit that works best for you, but you won't know for sure until you test other fruits you enjoy.

Ruti E.

For years, I've struggled with my weight. I've tried many diets. Some worked for a while, but I always regained the weight. When I participated in the Personalized Nutrition Project at the Weizmann Institute, I found out that tomatoes were causing me to have huge blood sugar spikes. Never in a million years would I have guessed that it was tomatoes! I sat down with one of the study coordinators after the study was over, and he showed me that in all my meals that included tomatoes, I had these obvious glucose spikes! The graphs were very clear and left no room for doubt. I have always eaten a lot of tomatoes, thinking I was doing myself a favor, but now I realize this could have been a major contributor to my previous diet failures. It wasn't my fault—it was the tomatoes! I have now significantly reduced my tomato intake and I'm feeling much more energetic, which still surprises me. I have already lost a couple of pounds, and I have high hopes that I have finally found the answer to my weight struggle, too.

- **Manipulate your juice.** Juice contains highly concentrated fruit sugar, but you might be able to drink a different juice without spiking your blood sugar. Freshly squeezed juice doesn't have the additives and the added sugars many packaged juices contain. The problem may also be the specific fruit. Swap out your orange juice for grapefruit juice, apple juice, or tomato juice, and see if those make a difference. You could also try eating a whole orange instead of drinking orange juice. This will provide more fiber, which could modify your blood sugar reaction. Another option is to eliminate the juice, if you don't care about it that much and drink it only out of habit. A glass of water might be preferable—in our research, we saw that more water with a meal tended to lower blood sugar reactions. Also, drinking water instead of a sweet beverage means you are consuming less energy, which can either help with weight loss or give you room to eat more food during the day.

- **Manipulate your added sugar.** If you always use cane sugar on your hot cereal, try a different added sugar, like honey, real maple syrup, coconut sugar, date sugar, or a little molasses. Or, if you have fruit in your oatmeal, maybe you would still like the taste without the added sugar.

- **Manipulate your milk.** Milk is a source of protein, calcium, and fat (except for nonfat milk), but what some people don't realize is that milk is also a source of carbohydrates because of the high levels of lactose (milk sugar) it contains. In fact, the more fat that is removed from natural milk, the more concentrated the natural milk sugar, so nonfat milk is the most "sugary." Even if you don't get a blood sugar rise from nonfat milk, you may find that adding higher-fat milk or cream to a meal that gives you a blood sugar spike might modify the spike. You could use 2 percent or whole milk, or even a splash of cream. You might also try soy milk, almond milk, or another nut or seed milk. You might react more favorably to a nut milk than a dairy milk, or vice versa.

When you try a different carb, simply test the meal again and put it into your chart (or into the app). Then you can compare the blood sugar rises (or hunger levels, if you are hunger tracking, or weekly weight changes) to see if the swap made any difference. If it lowered the rise in blood sugar to a level that is more characteristic for you, then you can add that food back in to your meals. If it didn't, you could try a different swap (or see if the other strategies offered on the following pages will work). How many times you will need to manipulate a meal probably depends on how much that meal means to you, but as you can see, there are many ways to manipulate the carbohydrates in any given meal. The trick is to find the manipulation that reduces your blood sugar spike without compromising your enjoyment of the meal.

ADD MORE FAT

Another powerful way you may be able to blunt your blood sugar spikes is to add fat. We have discussed the misconception that fat is bad, and when it comes to blood sugar, this seems to be quite true. In many cases, adding fat to a carbohydrate-rich food decreased the blood sugar spike, sometimes dramatically. You might be happy to hear this because fat tastes good and makes other foods taste better. If you have been avoiding it for your health, you may discover that you don't have to do that anymore.

There are many foods that are high in fat and easy to add to your meals:

- Animal fat, like lard
- Avocadoes
- Butter
- Cheese
- Coconut
- Cream
- Fatty meats, such as steak and bacon
- Mayonnaise
- Nuts and seeds (and nut and seed butters)
- Olive oil
- Peanuts and peanut butter
- Salmon and other fatty fish
- Tahini
- Whole eggs
- Whole milk

Just think of all the great ways you could make your meals tastier with added fat: a bit of butter on your toast, a touch of mayonnaise on your sandwich, olive oil on your pasta, tahini on your pita bread, cheese on your crackers, cream on your oatmeal, whole-milk café lattes…If you really would rather have prime rib than grilled chicken breast or you long for a whole-egg cheese omelet instead of that egg-white omelet you always force yourself to order, you may be pleasantly surprised how fat can keep your blood sugar in check. So, if you love a food and it spikes your blood sugar but doesn't already contain a lot of fat, or you've been eating low fat for your health but can't seem to control your blood sugar, see what happens when you add more fat. It may just bring that food right into your sweet spot. You could track your fat-adding experiment like this:

MEAL	30 min	60 min	90 min	120 min
Bagel, dry				
Bagel with butter				
Bagel with peanut butter				
Bagel with Nutella				

As you test, you will likely see that some fat additions may work better than others do, and some may cause a higher spike. You won't know until you test.

Should You Go Low Carb or Ketogenic?

After blood sugar testing, many people notice that they tend to have higher blood sugar spikes with high-carb foods and much lower blood sugar spikes with high-fat foods. This leads many to consider whether they should go on a low-carb, Paleo-style, or even ketogenic diet. The popularity of these various diets comes and goes, but they all have one thing in common: They are lower in carbohydrates and higher in fat than the standard American diet. As we discussed in the first half of this book, there is a lot of research that supports better, faster weight loss with low-carb diets than with low-fat diets. Diets like the Atkins diet and other similar programs have many followers. Recent versions of low-carb diets like the Paleo diet use many of the same principles, while also emphasizing whole natural foods over processed foods. Ketogenic diets take this to the extreme, with virtually no carbohydrates and very high fat levels. Traditionally, they have been used effectively to treat diseases, especially epilepsy in children. They have recently become more of a fad among people seeking to lose weight.

The research on the health benefits of these high-fat diets is somewhat mixed, although in general, there is no solid evidence they are dangerous. There is plenty of evidence that high-sugar diets are detrimental to health, so any of these diets would be an improvement over a high-sugar diet and would likely result in a very steady and low blood sugar level.

The problem is that these diets won't work well for everyone. Like anything else, the reactions people have to these diets are personalized. If you want to try going low carb / high fat, then go ahead, but be sure to test your blood sugar as you try different meals to see what is working for you that you actually like to eat.

Another problem with these diets is compliance. It is very difficult to be low carb in our society today. Think of all the places you go and things that you do, and imagine never being able to eat carbs in all those situations. It's very difficult to attend social events or eat at restaurants without eating carbs. Carbs are everywhere; they are tempting, and tasty, and many people who go low carb or ketogenic discover that they can't keep it up for very long. Carb cravings may disappear at first but then may resurface and be irresistible. Many people report that once they go back to carb-rich foods, they overeat them and regain any lost weight.

It is up to you, but we would say that if you like to eat a low-carb diet and don't have a problem sticking with it, and you also make sure your diet is varied and balanced with plenty of vitamins and minerals, then it could be a great diet for you. But if you don't like eating that way, and especially for a long period of time, we don't recommend it, because you probably won't stick to it. It will feel too restrictive. If you like carbs, then find out which ones don't cause blood sugar problems, then enjoy them without guilt.

GO NATURAL

Many processed foods contain food additives that tend to spike blood sugar in many people. The most obvious is artificial sweeteners, which we have talked about at length and may spike blood sugar in some consumers. In such susceptible individuals, such processed foods may affect glucose intolerance in general and contribute to the development of diabetes (although more research in humans is needed). But there are many other examples of how processed and packaged food can spike blood sugar.

For example, we have a friend who loved to drive through a popular chain restaurant and order their breakfast sandwiches. She often got the low-fat, "healthy" versions with egg white and turkey bacon on whole-grain English muffins, but sometimes she got the fattier versions as well. In all cases, she had a blood sugar spike—it didn't seem to matter if she added butter or cheese or meat or if she went with egg whites and no fat. What she did notice was that if she made a breakfast sandwich at home just the way she liked it, with whole eggs, bacon, and cheese, she would get a much lower blood sugar spike. As an experiment, she tried a whole-grain sandwich with egg white and turkey sausage at home and also did not get a blood sugar spike.

We suspect it was the preservatives and other additives in the drive-through food that were the cause of the spike. Many of the carbohydrate-based products in fast food and other restaurants are made with highly processed ingredients, and the sauces and flavorings added to the food often contain sugar and a very high amount of sodium, even if they don't taste sweet or overly salty. Both could influence blood sugar spikes.

Many processed foods have removed the fat and consider this a point of pride, but to remove fat and retain a good flavor, sugar and additives often fill in. Artificial coloring and flavoring also tends to promote blood sugar instability, so if you absolutely must have a particular packaged food, see if you can use the strategies in this chapter to manipulate it so it works for you. If not, try substituting something similar that you make at home, like that breakfast sandwich our friend likes, or try a more natural version of a favorite food, like an ice-cream bar with a shorter ingredients list.

Doron P.

I've been dieting all my life. I'm in the hi-tech industry and I work crazy hours, and have for many years. The stress in my life made me unable to endure the highly restrictive nature of most diets and the feeling of hunger I always get. I just can't resist the good foods that are so easy to eat in my work environment. But now I'm in my midforties and I must concede that my lifelong weight-loss efforts aren't working. I was beginning to wonder if I was destined to be obese and suffer the complications so common with this problem. Then I enrolled in the Personalized Nutrition Project. I felt like this could be my last chance. When I got my report, I was surprised to see that several of the "healthy foods" I was eating, like sushi, fruit salad, and my favorite eggplant dish, were in fact not good for my blood sugar levels at all. Other unexpected foods, like wine, chocolate, and crème brûlée, hardly affected my blood sugar levels. For the first time in my life, I could self-construct a balanced diet based on me. I can now eat with some reassurance, and the occasional desserts that agree with me. This helps me adhere to a plan because it is not overly restrictive and includes foods I love that feel indulgent. I am feeling great, and after two years of following the diet, I have lost almost 20 pounds!

LIFESTYLE MANIPULATION

In addition to changing the foods you eat, there are lifestyle changes that can influence blood sugar spikes one way or another. We won't cover variables that you can't control daily, like age, weight, BMI, or measures like waking blood sugar, cholesterol level, blood pressure, or HbA1c percentage. But there are some other things that you can change daily (or as needed), and you can play around with them to see if they modify your spikes in a positive way.

- **Sleep more.** In our study, we observed that more sleep resulted in lower postmeal blood sugar responses. Specifically, sleep coinciding with nighttime was more conducive to lower responses than sleeping during the day and being awake at night. If you don't currently get enough sleep (general guidelines say you should get 7 to 8 hours, but this may vary for you), see if increasing your sleep or adjusting your sleep hours has an impact on the blood sugar spikes you see after eating your favorite meals.
- **Exercise more.** In general, in our research we found an association between exercise and lower blood glucose

levels, evidence that being physically active can be a useful manipulation that can broadly affect your glucose responses. Again, this doesn't work for everyone, so we will only say that you can test to see whether it affects your personal levels or not. Sometimes, the exercise effect was immediate, and sometimes, we found it did not kick in for 24 hours, so keep this in mind when you test for yourself.

- **Adjust meal timing.** There are many variations in how individuals react to meal timing. Many people have higher blood sugar spikes in the morning and lower spikes in the evening; others notice the opposite trend. You may find that eating foods that spike blood sugar at a different time of day can blunt the spike. Try your favorite breakfast as an afternoon snack, or try your late-night spiking snack as a component of your midday lunch, to see if that makes a difference.

- **Less salt, more water.** For some people, salty foods caused higher postmeal blood sugar responses, and more water with the meal caused lower postmeal blood sugar responses. You could try adjusting salt and water in your meal to see if that helps.

- **Consider your hormonal shifts.** Women who were menstruating tended to have more blood sugar spikes than they did at other times during their cycle. You may not want to do your one week of food tests when you are menstruating, because the results may not be accurate. Or, you may want to take even more precautions with your food choices during that week, reducing carbohydrates and adding fat in a way that keeps blood sugar lower.

- **Try relaxation.** Our research showed an association between stress and higher blood glucose levels, so if you have been going through a stressful time, your levels may be higher than they would be otherwise. It may be useful to practice stress management techniques like deep breathing, relaxation exercises, or meditation. If you want to try these, you can test your blood sugar to see if it helps. We have seen it make a difference in some cases.

Ron K.

After taking part in the Weizmann study on personalized nutrition, which included a continuous glucose monitor I wore all the time, I found out that whenever I eat late at night, my blood glucose levels are all over the place all through the night. The following morning, I wake up with high blood glucose levels. I decided to pay much more attention to what I eat before going to sleep and specifically choose different foods to eat late at night. I also experimented with not eating so late, moving my last meal earlier. I couldn't always do this, but I tried. After the study, I could only test with finger-pricking, so I couldn't be sure what my blood sugar was doing at night, but I did realize that certain changes in food choices and timing made me feel much better in the morning, and my fasting glucose level after waking up began to stay lower on a more regular basis. I consider that a success!

Finally, if you have tried several different strategies and a particular meal or food continues to spike your blood sugar, it may be best to phase that meal or food out of your diet. Some foods are going to spike some people no matter what, and it is worth taking that food out, or at least not eating it as often, for the sake your health, energy, weight, and general well-being. That food just isn't right for you. If this seems difficult or you don't like this idea, just remember how important it is to maintain normal blood sugar levels after eating. This will benefit your health and weight in many ways. Eventually you may lose your taste for it and come to prefer other foods with more favorable effects. This is what a personalized diet is really all about. Now you know the truth, for you. That means it's time to get your personalized food plan and lifestyle organized!

CHAPTER 10

Your Personalized Diet Organizer

After our research study was over, we realized we could not just move on to our next project and leave our study subjects without further guidance. People wanted to know what to do with the information they had discovered during the study. They had their lists of good and bad foods, but they weren't sure what to do with them. How were they supposed to organize their meals, knowing what they had learned? They wanted a plan. We spent a lot of time thinking about this. What considerations would have to go into the building of a complete meal plan based on blood sugar results? How could we help?

The first thing we did was to consider what must go into any solid meal plan. Of course, a primary goal is to maintain stable, normal blood sugar levels. There are some additional important considerations for a sound, healthful diet. If you want to regain or maintain good health and healthy body weight, it would be wise to do the following:

- **Eat a wide variety of foods.** If your tests revealed a small group of meals that don't spike your blood sugar, that's great information, but if you eat only those few meals, you probably won't get the full range of nutrients you need. It's beyond the scope of this book to tell you the proper intake of every macronutrient, vitamin, and mineral you require, and that likely varies by person anyway, but the best way to get a wide range of nutrients is to eat a wide variety of foods. That means different types of vegetables, fruits, grains, and protein sources. Or, more simply, it means different types of meals—eggs, soups, salads, sandwiches, protein/vegetable plates, pasta/rice dishes, and so on. If you vary the foods you eat, it will likely benefit your nutrient intake. In the meal plan later in this chapter, we will help you categorize your "good" meals to be sure you are getting a variety of food in your diet. You don't have to eat every kind of meal every day, or ever—if you don't like soup or you're not a sandwich person, that's completely fine, but the more variety you get in your meal types, the more nutrients you are likely to get, too. If your tested "good" meals don't provide a range (or even if they do), we strongly encourage you to continue to diversify your diet, trying new things and testing new meals you enjoy. Continue adding to your list of "good" meals and foods, and you will have an increasingly long list of safe options that will nourish you and keep your blood sugar under control.
- **Include fiber.** Remember that fiber feeds your good microbiome bacteria and can increase their diversity.

Vegetables, fruits, grains, seeds, and fiber supplements are all good sources of fiber, to keep your microbiome well fed and thriving. Also remember that although fiber may lead to higher blood sugar levels initially, it tends to bring down blood sugar levels the next day. Regular fiber intake can help you keep your blood sugar levels stable.

- **Balance your portions.** You may have already experimented with portion sizes when working to manipulate some of your blood sugar spikes so that they trend downward. As we've already explained, eating too much, even of foods that do not spike your blood sugar when eaten in moderation, can cause blood sugar spikes in some people. Regularly overeating can also mean you are taking in more energy (calories) than you need, and over time, this will almost certainly result in weight gain.

When your blood sugar levels are stable, you will be more likely to maintain your weight while eating more calories than you would on a calorie-reduction diet that doesn't take blood sugar into consideration. Remember the study that demonstrated that people eating a low-carb diet could lose just as much weight as people eating a low-fat diet, while taking in more calories? The reason for the difference is likely the blood sugar effect because the postspike insulin rise is well known to contribute to fat storage. So, while you can probably eat more and stay satiated when your blood sugar levels stay in check, there are limits.

Of course, there are occasions when you need to eat large meals. You will be hungrier at some times than at others, and then of course there are celebrations, family dinners, and restaurant meals, all of which tend to have servings on the large side.

It is very useful to know, from your testing, which large meals don't spike your blood sugar. If there is an 800-calorie meal that doesn't spike you, then you can fall back on that when you need more energy. Even better, find several that work for you or that work after manipulating certain aspects (like carb swapping and/or adding fat). If you are trying to lose weight, then you can work on reducing portion sizes to the point where you don't feel hungry but are still losing weight slowly and steadily. Remember, keeping your blood sugar level will allow you to eat more and maintain an energy deficit. There is no way for us (or anyone) to tell you that a certain number of calories will result in weight loss *for you*. You need to find that level at which you start losing weight, so focus on finding the best blood-sugar-stabilizing foods for you, eating as much diversity as possible within that parameter, and eating those foods in moderate portions.

Another way to help you control your food intake, either for weight loss or to prevent weight gain, is by organizing your "good" meals into large (more than 500 calories), moderate (200 to 500 calories), and small (fewer than 200 calories) meals/snacks, and balancing these throughout the day. You can choose to stick with moderate meals and small snacks, or balance large meals and small meals throughout the day (or week). This approach should work quite well and doesn't require counting calories. Remember, if you don't have enough "good" choices in any category, you can continue to test to find more options. We recommend always seeking more dietary diversity.

MY *GOOD* FOODS AND MEALS

The next step is to create a master list of all the meals and foods that you checked as "good" on the chart on page 258. This will serve as your personalized diet menu, and it is from this list that you will choose the foods you eat on a daily basis. Include the meals and foods that did not initially give you a blood sugar spike or that you were able to modify to eliminate an initial blood sugar spike.

My Good Foods and Meals
Breakfast:
Lunch:
Dinner:
Snacks:
Miscellaneous Foods:

Now that you have all your "good" foods organized, you can create your meal plan. This should be completely individual to you, considering what you like; how often you like to eat; how much food you need; and other factors, including what foods are in season, your budget, and so on. Use your "Good Food" list as your master guide.

Of course, there will be times when you can't follow your plan. Life happens and you will need to be flexible, and when the unexpected occurs (or the scheduled social event, outing, or vacation), you will already have the tools to face that situation and make good choices. Fill out your plan based on all the "good" meals and snacks you have already organized. Most importantly, remember to do the following:

- **Keep your choices diverse.** The more variety in the things you eat, the more nutrients you will get. Try mixing up different food types (e.g., soup, salad, grain-based dishes, protein-based dishes, etc.).
- **Keep your portions balanced.** Stay moderate, or balance large meals with small meals.
- **Keep experimenting!** The world is filled with thousands of different foods, and they can be grouped into endless combinations that might be good for you, enjoyable, and blood sugar stabilizing. Keep testing, keep trying new things, and be a food adventurer, but let the foundation of your diet be those meals and foods that keep your blood sugar stable and steady. This is how you will find dietary freedom at last.

	Breakfast	Lunch	Dinner	Snacks
M				
T				
W				
Th				
F				
Sa				
Su				

We suggest copying this template and printing one out each week to fill out, for your guidance. You can either fill it out at the beginning of the week, before you go shopping, to have a plan, or you can fill it out after you eat each meal, to be sure you are staying on course.

Once you get used to planning your meals in this way, you probably won't need to continue to write out the plans, although some people prefer to do this regularly, just to stay organized and to remind themselves what is and is not best for them to eat. We also recommend retesting foods you eat often every six months or so. As your diet shifts, your microbiome will shift, too, and over time, your reactions to certain foods may change. The changes probably won't be dramatic, but you might find some foods that you couldn't eat before will become acceptable.

The essence of the personalized diet is, of course, that it is all about you, so we hope you will resist the temptation to lapse back into traditional diets and instead remain curious and committed to your own personal reactions to foods. Continue testing your blood sugar response to foods as you go forward and trying new things frequently to expand your dietary horizons and food diversity and to encourage your own quest for better health.

CHAPTER 11

The Future of Dieting

You are now a part of the revolution-in-motion in nutrition science. You are practicing personalized nutrition, using information on the forefront of human knowledge, and putting into practice science that has yet to be incorporated into mainstream dietary guidance. There is still much to know and much to learn, and there is certainly much to anticipate. In this final chapter, we want to give you a glimpse into the future so you can see what's already in development, what's coming next, and what you have to look forward to, in terms of new research knowledge and new technologies that will make personalized dieting not just easier but also increasingly personalized.

For example, as we learn how better to design personalized nutrition programs, there are many other measures beyond blood sugar to consider. Eventually there will probably be easy ways to track blood lipid fluctuations (cholesterol levels), blood pressure changes, and more detailed and periodic monitoring of the microbiome, including direct intervention to improve microbiome configuration and function. Getting individual metrics using sensors and "big data" approaches like those that we have used in our blood glucose research will yield more information in the near future. Also, personalization related to genetics is in its infancy, and we can expect much more to come from research into this field.

Major food companies are also looking at the possibilities of personalizing food in the future. For example, Nestlé is working on a machine, similar to a Nespresso machine, that makes espresso from capsules that can customize a food, beverage, or supplement for the individual, at the push of a button, based on your individual nutrient deficiencies and requirements.[1]

Another exciting area of development is in technological advancements for tracking your own biometrics. There are many new wearables and sensors that can track health measures like pulse, heart rate, blood sugar, and more. Soon there may even be a device for measuring microbiome composition at home. All this new technology will become an important tool in advancing the consumer's awareness of how individual bodies respond to food and lifestyle decisions.

Some of these advancements are still in the speculation stage, but the following are a few technologies we know are deep in development or are recently available that could enhance your personalized diet now or soon.

NONINVASIVE CONTINUOUS BLOOD GLUCOSE MONITORS

There are continuous blood glucose monitors that do not require finger pricking. A company called Abbott just came out with one called Libre Pro. The old monitors required calibration finger pricking four times a day. Newer models are termed "minimally invasive" because they require a tiny insertion of a miniature needle into the skin but does not require finger pricking for continuous calibration. A reader costs around $80 and can be used multiple times. A sensor costs around $80 and can be used once for a period of two weeks, after which it must be replaced with another sensor. The problem is that currently, these monitors are available only by prescription for people who have been diagnosed with diabetes, but at least one consumer company is working on producing a similar product to target the general population. We believe that as demand increases with more people monitoring their own blood sugar without having a diabetes diagnosis that these devices will become available to anyone, and the prices will come down.

MICROBIOME ANALYSIS

After our study was completed, the Weizmann Institute of Science (our research institute) licensed our algorithm to a start-up company called DayTwo (which did not fund our study). Day-Two can analyze stool samples and provide a complete report on microbiome composition. The company takes the microbiome information and uses our algorithm to predict how the person providing the sample will respond to different foods and meals. The main difference between this method and blood sugar testing is that DayTwo uses advanced data based on microbiome content from a stool sample to *predict* how you will respond to meals. No blood sugar testing necessary. While explaining the exact nature and content of these algorithms is beyond the scope of this book, suffice it to say that the DayTwo product integrates a highly detailed microbiome characterization and a gigantic database of biometric information collected from thousands of people to generate its highly accurate predictions of personalized responses to individual foods, food combinations, and diverse meals. The results you can get from this company are quite powerful.

But of course, you don't have to buy this product. Blood sugar testing, as explained in this book, takes more time but it does give you a direct, easy, accessible way to see your immediate response to the specific meals you actually eat. Still, we expect many readers will likely be interested in this test, so you can find out more at www.daytwo.com.

WEARABLE SENSORS

We are seeing more hi-tech companies developing self-monitoring devices of various kinds. Many are already available. Some monitor number of steps, calories burned, and heart rate (like Fitbit and Apple Watch), and each new release seems to add more features, like sleep tracking and blood pressure. These wearables give you information, although they don't give you advice about what to do with it. In the medical field, there are more wearables that we expect will eventually trickle down into the general population—devices for monitoring heart irregularities, brain activity, muscle activity, body temperature, sleep apnea, sweat rate, as well as activity related to stress and mental disturbance.[2]

Someday (and we believe sooner rather than later), these technologies could help general consumers monitor their own health and catch or arrest disease processes earlier, as well as monitor the relative success of dietary and other lifestyle interventions.

"OMICS" APPROACHES

One of the most exciting revolutions occurring in science and medicine includes the use of advanced computational platforms that are now able to analyze endless quantities of individualized big data and apply them to multiple facets and aspects of human health and disease. Some examples are the sequencing of the human genome (genomics) and measuring levels of gut bacteria (microbiomics), bacterial product levels (metabolics), and gene activity by RNA level (transcriptomics). Other examples include comprehensive blood tests and sequences of various imaging measures. These new capabilities, which just a few years ago were regarded as science fiction, now enable us to analyze the human body with unprecedented precision and accuracy.

Some companies are already offering a subset of these (e.g., only human genomes or only gut bacteria), while others have loftier goals with more extensive evaluations. Right now, the state of this art is still at the measurement phase, and the data coming out has not been clearly linked to actions people can take based on the information. We expect that as more data accumulates, there will be more obvious recommendations that can be gleaned from it, which could potentially benefit individuals. That will take time and the kind of extensive research we have done with blood sugar to prove a positive effect of any action advice, but if and when this is accomplished, the potential to reduce disease incidence, improve health, and tailor individualized treatments for people based on their measurements will be one of the major directions in medicine and science. Someday perhaps soon, anyone will be able to get detailed molecular profiling that will result in a tailored approach to health and wellness.

As you can see, we are entering an era of massive data collection and analysis. Behavior, lifestyle, nutrition, genetics, the microbiome, and molecular data may all soon converge with information we already have about disease incidence and the onset of clinical markers for many different health conditions. The analysis of this data will eventually allow us to learn the "rules" of the human body and create more predictive algorithms for many different situations and settings. Someday, perhaps sooner than we think, we may each carry on us or within us an automated "doctor," perhaps in the form of an app or a wearable or even an implant, that will constantly take measurements and information about us and alert us before any negative health situation can develop. It could warn us *before* a heart attack or stroke, before cancer is incurable, even before obesity gets under way or becomes difficult to control. That day is not far away, and what we know right now, today, about blood sugar and personalized nutrition is just one more step in that direction.

Throughout this book, we've mentioned many people, including friends, colleagues, and the people in our research study, whose lives have been changed by personalizing their diets based on their blood sugar responses. Only time will tell whether personalized nutrition will change the course of the obesity epidemic and the rise of metabolic diseases, but we certainly hope that it will turn this trend around and send human health back in the right direction. If personalized nutrition indeed marks the beginning of a change in the way we view our own health, lifestyle, and food choices, then we are happy to contribute to it, and we welcome you as fellow participants to join in this paradigm shift. As your health improves, so improves the health of our world.

NOTES

Introduction: Welcome to the Future of Dieting

1. M. Bergman et al. "One-Hour Post-Load Plasma Glucose Level during the OGTT Predicts Mortality: Observations from the Israel Study of Glucose Intolerance, Obesity and Hypertension." *Epidemiology* 33, no. 8 (2016): 1060–1066. http://onlinelibrary.wiley.com/doi/10.1111/dme.13116/abstract.

Chapter 1: A Bread Story

1. A. Aubrey and M. Godoy. "75 Percent of Americans Say They Eat Healthy—Despite Evidence to the Contrary." The Salt: NPR.org. August 3, 2016. http://www.npr.org/sections/thesalt/2016/08/03/487640479/75-percent-of-americans-say-they-eat-healthy-despite-evidence-to-the-contrary.

2. FAOSTAT statistics database. *Food and Agriculture Organization of the United Nations*, 1998.

3. D. Zeevi et al. "Personalized Nutrition by Prediction of Glycemic Responses." *Cell* 163, no. 5 (2015): 1079–1094. http://www.cell.com/abstract/S0092-8674(15)01481-6.

4. F. Salamini et al. "Genetics and Geography of Wild Cereal Domestication in the Near East." *Nature Reviews Genetics* 3 (2002): 429–441. http://www.nature.com/nrg/journal/v3/n6/full/nrg817.html.

5. J. L. Slavin et al. "The Role of Whole Grains in Disease Prevention." *Journal of the American Dietetic Association* 101, no. 7 (2001): 780–785. https://www.ncbi.nlm.nih.gov/pubmed/11478475.

6. Ibid.

7. C. A. Batt and M. Tortorelo. "Encyclopedia of Food Microbiology." Academic Press, June 10, 2014.

8. F. Minervini et al. "Ecological Parameters Influencing Microbial Diversity and Stability of Traditional Sourdough." *International Journal of Food Microbiology* 171 (2014): 136–146. https://www.ncbi.nlm.nih.gov /pubmed/24355817.

9. E. K. Arendt et al. "Impact of Sourdough on the Texture of Bread." *Food Microbiology* 24, no. 2 (2007): 165–174. http://www.sciencedirect.com /science/article/pii/S0740002006001614.

10. M. Bach Kristensen et al. "A Decrease in Iron Status in Young Healthy Women after Long-Term Daily Consumption of the Recommended Intake of Fibre-Rich Wheat Bread." *European Journal of Nutrition* 44, no. 6 (2005): 334–340. https://www.ncbi.nlm.nih.gov/pubmed/15349738.

11. D. Aune et al. "Whole Grain Consumption and Risk of Cardiovascular Disease, Cancer, and All Cause and Cause Specific Mortality: Systematic Review and Dose-Response Meta-Analysis of Prospective Studies." *British Medical Journal* 2016: 353. http://www.bmj.com/content/353/bmj.i2716.

12. D. R. Jacobs et al. "Whole-Grain Intake and Cancer: An Expanded Review and Meta-Analysis." *Nutrition and Cancer* 30, no. 2 (1998): 85–96. https://www.ncbi.nlm.nih.gov/pubmed/9589426.

13. P. B. Mellen et al. "Whole Grain Intake and Cardiovascular Disease: A Meta-Analysis." *Nutrition, Metabolism, and Cardiovascular Diseases* 18, no. 4 (2008): 283–290. https://www.ncbi.nlm.nih.gov/pubmed/17449231.

14. J. S. L. de Munter et al. "Whole Grain, Bran, and Germ Intake and Risk of Type 2 Diabetes: A Prospective Cohort Study and Systematic Review." *PLoS Medicine.* August 28, 2007. http://journals.plos.org/plosmedicine /article?id=10.1371/journal.pmed.0040261.

15. P. L. Lutsey et al. "Whole Grain Intake and Its Cross-Sectional Association with Obesity, Insulin Resistance, Inflammation, Diabetes and Subclinical CVD: The MESA Study." *British Journal of Nutrition* 98, no. 2 (2007): 397–405. https://www.ncbi.nlm.nih.gov/pubmed/17391554.

16. M. A. Pereira et al. "Effect of Whole Grains on Insulin Sensitivity in Overweight Hyperinsulinemic Adults." *American Journal of Clinical Nutrition* 75, no. 5 (2002): 848–855. https://www.ncbi.nlm.nih.gov/pubmed /11976158.

17. R. Giacco et al. "Effects of the Regular Consumption of Wholemeal Wheat Foods on Cardiovascular Risk Factors in Healthy People." *Nutrition, Metabolism, and Cardiovascular Diseases* 20, no. 3 (2010): 186–194. https:// www.ncbi.nlm.nih.gov/pubmed/19502018.

18. P. Tighe et al. "Effect of Increased Consumption of Whole-Grain Foods on Blood Pressure and Other Cardiovascular Risk Markers in Healthy Middle-Aged Persons: A Randomized Controlled Trial." *American Journal of*

Clinical Nutrition 92, no. 4 (2010): 733–740. https://www.ncbi.nlm.nih.gov /pubmed/20685951.

19. H. I. Katcher et al. "The Effects of a Whole Grain–Enriched Hypocaloric Diet on Cardiovascular Disease Risk Factors in Men and Women with Metabolic Syndrome." *American Journal of Clinical Nutrition* 87, no. 1 (2008): 79–90. http://ajcn.nutrition.org/content/87/1/79.full.

20. J. Montonen et al. "Consumption of Red Meat and Whole-Grain Bread in Relation to Biomarkers of Obesity, Inflammation, Glucose Metabolism and Oxidative Stress." *European Journal of Nutrition* 52, no. 1 (2013): 337–345. https://www.ncbi.nlm.nih.gov/pubmed/22426755.

21. R. Giacco et al. "Effects of the Regular Consumption of Wholemeal Wheat Foods on Cardiovascular Risk Factors in Healthy People." *Nutrition, Metabolism, and Cardiovascular Diseases* 20, no. 3 (2010): 186–194. https:// www.ncbi.nlm.nih.gov/pubmed/19502018.

22. M. K. Jensen et al. "Whole Grains, Bran, and Germ in Relation to Homocysteine and Markers of Glycemic Control, Lipids, and Inflammation 1." *American Journal of Clinical Nutrition* 83, no. 2 (2006): 275–283. https:// www.ncbi.nlm.nih.gov/pubmed/16469984.

23. F. Sofi et al. "Effects of Short-Term Consumption of Bread Obtained by an Old Italian Grain Variety on Lipid, Inflammatory, and Hemorheological Variables: An Intervention Study." *Journal of Medicinal Food* 13, no. 3 (2010): 615–620. https://www.ncbi.nlm.nih.gov/pubmed/20438321.

24. P. Tighe et al. "Effect of Increased Consumption of Whole-Grain Foods on Blood Pressure and Other Cardiovascular Risk Markers in Healthy Middle-Aged Persons: A Randomized Controlled Trial." *American Journal of Clinical Nutrition* 92, no. 4 (2010): 733–740. https://www.ncbi.nlm.nih.gov /pubmed/20685951.

25. P. Vitaglione et al. "Whole-Grain Wheat Consumption Reduces Inflammation in a Randomized Controlled Trial on Overweight and Obese Subjects with Unhealthy Dietary and Lifestyle Behaviors: Role of Polyphenols Bound to Cereal Dietary Fiber." *American Journal of Clinical Nutrition* 101, no. 2 (2015): 251–261. https://www.ncbi.nlm.nih.gov/pubmed/25646321.

26. A. Andersson et al. "Whole-Grain Foods Do Not Affect Insulin Sensitivity or Markers of Lipid Peroxidation and Inflammation in Healthy, Moderately Overweight Subjects." *Journal of Nutrition* 137, no. 6 (2007): 1401–1407. https://www.ncbi.nlm.nih.gov/pubmed/17513398.

27. I. A. Brownlee et al. "Markers of Cardiovascular Risk Are Not Changed by Increased Whole-Grain Intake: The WHOLEheart Study, a Randomised, Controlled Dietary Intervention." *British Journal of Nutrition* 104, no. 1 (2010): 125–134. https://www.ncbi.nlm.nih.gov/pubmed/20307353.

28. A. Costabile et al. "Whole-Grain Wheat Breakfast Cereal Has a Prebiotic Effect on the Human Gut Microbiota: A Double-Blind, Placebo-Controlled, Crossover Study." *British Journal of Nutrition* 99, no. 1 (2008): 110–120. https://www.ncbi.nlm.nih.gov/pubmed/17761020.

29. R. Giacco et al. "Effects of the Regular Consumption of Wholemeal Wheat Foods on Cardiovascular Risk Factors in Healthy People." *Nutrition, Metabolism, and Cardiovascular Diseases* 20, no. 3 (2010): 186–194. https://www.ncbi.nlm.nih.gov/pubmed/19502018.

30. A. J. Tucker et al. "The Effect of Whole Grain Wheat Sourdough Bread Consumption on Serum Lipids in Healthy Normoglycemic/Normoinsulinemic and Hyperglycemic/Hyperinsulinemic Adults Depends on Presence of the APOE E3/E3 Genotype: A Randomized Controlled Trial." *Nutrition & Metabolism* 7, no. 37 (2010). https://www.ncbi.nlm.nih.gov/pubmed/20444273.

31. B. Chassaing et al. "Dietary Emulsifiers Impact the Mouse Gut Microbiota Promoting Colitis and Metabolic Syndrome." *Nature* 519, no. 7541 (2015): 92–96. https://www.ncbi.nlm.nih.gov/pubmed/25731162.

32. J. Lappi et al. "Sourdough Fermentation of Wholemeal Wheat Bread Increases Solubility of Arabinoxylan and Protein and Decreases Postprandial Glucose and Insulin Responses." *Journal of Cereal Science* 51, no. 1 (2010): 152–158. http://www.sciencedirect.com/science/article/pii/S0733521009001738.

33. K. Poutanen et al. "Sourdough and Cereal Fermentation in a Nutritional Perspective." *Food Microbiology* 26, no. 7 (2009): 693–699. https://www.ncbi.nlm.nih.gov/pubmed/19747602.

Chapter 2: Modern (Health) Problems

1. "Achievements in Public Health, 1900–1999: Control of Infectious Diseases." *Morbidity and Mortality Weekly Report, Centers for Disease Control and Prevention* 48, no. 29 (1999): 621–629. http://www.cdc.gov/mmwR/preview/mmwrhtml/mm4829a1.htm.

2. H. A. Coller. "Is Cancer a Metabolic Disease?" *American Journal of Pathology* 184, no. 1 (2014): 4–17. http://ajp.amjpathol.org/article/S0002-9440(13)00653-6/fulltext.

3. H. Cai et al. "Metabolic Dysfunction in Alzheimer's Disease and Related Neurodegenerative Disorders." *Current Alzheimer Research* 9, no. 1 (2012): 5–17. https://www.ncbi.nlm.nih.gov/pubmed/22329649.

4. P. Zhang and B. Tian. "Metabolic Syndrome: An Important Risk Factor for Parkinson's Disease." *Oxidative Medicine and Cellular Longevity* 2014, article ID 729194. https://www.hindawi.com/journals/omcl/2014/729194/cta.

5. P. Paschos and K. Paletas. "Non Alcoholic Fatty Liver Disease and Metabolic Syndrome." *Hippokratia* 13, no. 1 (2009): 9–19. https://www.ncbi.nlm.nih.gov /pmc/articles/PMC2633261.

6. "Overweight & Obesity Statistics." National Institute of Diabetes and Digestive and Kidney Diseases, October 2012. https://www.niddk.nih .gov/health-information/health-statistics/Pages/overweight-obesity-statistics .aspx#top.

7. "Obesity and Overweight Fact Sheet." World Health Organization, June 2016. http://www.who.int/mediacentre/factsheets/fs311/en.

8. "Diabetes Fact Sheet." World Health Organization, July 2017. http:// www.who.int/mediacentre/factsheets/fs312/en.

9. "Diabetes Latest." Centers for Disease Control and Prevention, June 2014. https://www.cdc.gov/features/diabetesfactsheet.

10. "Heart Disease, Stroke and Research Statistics At-a-Glance." American Heart Association, American Stroke Association, December 2015. http:// www.heart.org/idc/groups/ahamah-public/@wcm/@sop/@smd/documents /downloadable/ucm_480086.pdf.

11. J. Worland. "More Than a Third of U.S. Adults Have Metabolic Syndrome." *Time Health*, May 19, 2015. http://time.com/3887131/metabolic -syndrome-obesity.

12. "Cancer Facts & Figures 2017." American Cancer Society, 2017. https://www.cancer.org/content/dam/cancer-org/research/cancer-facts-and -statistics/annual-cancer-facts-and-figures/2017/cancer-facts-and-figures -2017.pdf.

13. "Heart Disease and Stroke Statistics—At-a-Glance." American Heart Association, American Stroke Association, 2015. https://www.heart.org /idc/groups/ahamah-public/@wcm/@sop/@smd/documents/downloadable /ucm_470704.pdf.

14. M. Ahmed. "Non-alcoholic Fatty Liver Disease in 2015." *World Journal of Hepatology* 7, no. 11 (2015): 1450–1459. https://www.ncbi.nlm.nih .gov/pmc/articles/PMC4462685.

15. "Liver Disease: The Big Picture." American Liver Foundation, October 2013. http://www.liverfoundation.org/education/liverlowdown/ll1013 /bigpicture.

16. "2017 Alzheimer's Disease Facts and Figures." Alzheimer's Association, 2017. http://www.alz.org/facts.

17. "Parkinson's Disease Q&A." Parkinson's Disease Foundation, 2016. http://www.pdf.org/pdf/pubs_parkinson_qa_16.pdf.

18. "Long-Term Trends in Diabetes." Centers for Disease Control and Prevention, Division of Diabetes Translation, April 2016. https://www.cdc.gov /diabetes/statistics/slides/long_term_trends.pdf.

19. "Four-Decade Study: Americans Taller, Fatter." Live Science, October 27, 2004. http://www.livescience.com/49-decade-study-americans-taller-fatter.html.

20. R. Dotinga. "The Average Americans' Weight Change since the 1980s Is Startling." CBS News, August 3, 2016. http://www.cbsnews.com/news/americans-weight-gain-since-1980s-startling.

21. "Life Expectancy Increases Globally as Death Toll Falls from Major Diseases." Institute for Health Metrics and Evaluation, 2014. http://www.healthdata.org/news-release/life-expectancy-increases-globally-death-toll-falls-major-diseases.

22. V. Dengler et al. "Disruption of Circadian Rhythms and Sleep in Critical Illness and Its Impact on Innate Immunity." *Current Pharmaceutical Design* 21, no. 24 (2015): 3469–3476. https://www.ncbi.nlm.nih.gov/pubmed/26144943.

23. T. Eckle. "Health Impact and Management of a Disrupted Circadian Rhythm and Sleep in Critical Illnesses." *Current Pharmaceutical Design* 21, no. 24 (2015): 3428–3430. https://www.ncbi.nlm.nih.gov/pmc/articles/PMC4673005/#R9.

24. U. Schibler. "The Daily Rhythms of Genes, Cells and Organs." *EMBO Reports* 6, S1 (2005): S67–S62. http://embor.embopress.org/content/6/S1/S9.

25. A. J. Lewy et al. "Light Suppresses Melatonin Secretion in Humans." *Science* 210, no. 4475 (1980): 1267–1269. https://www.ncbi.nlm.nih.gov/pubmed/7434030.

26. K. Wulff et al. "Sleep and Circadian Rhythm Disruption in Psychiatric and Neurodegenerative Disease." *Nature Reviews Neuroscience* 11 (2010): 589–599. http://www.nature.com/nrn/journal/v11/n8/full/nrn2868.html.

27. R. B. Costello et al. "The Effectiveness of Melatonin for Promoting Healthy Sleep: A Rapid Evidence Assessment of the Literature." *Nutrition Journal* 13, no. 106 (2014). https://www.ncbi.nlm.nih.gov/pmc/articles/PMC4273450/.

28. A. Grundy et al. "Shift Work, Circadian Gene Variants and Risk of Breast Cancer." *Cancer Epidemiology* 37, no. 5 (2013): 606–612. https://www.ncbi.nlm.nih.gov/pubmed/23725643.

29. F. C. Kelleher et al. "Circadian Molecular Clocks and Cancer." *Cancer Letters* 342, no. 1 (2014): 9–18. https:www.ncbi.nlm.nih.gov/pubmed/24099911.

30. R. G. Stevens. "Circadian Disruption and Breast Cancer: From Melatonin to Clock Genes." *Epidemiology* 16, no. 2 (2005): 254–258. http://journals.lww.com/epidem/Abstract/2005/03000/Circadian_Disruption_and_Breast_Cancer__From.16.aspx.

31. K. Wulff et al. "Sleep and Circadian Rhythm Disruption in Psychiatric and Neurodegenerative Disease." *Nature Reviews Neuroscience* 11, no. 8 (2010): 589–599. https://www.ncbi.nlm.nih.gov/pubmed/20631712.

32. J. Emens et al. "Circadian Misalignment in Major Depressive Disorder." *Psychiatry Research* 168, no. 3 (2009): 259–261. http://www.psy-journal .com/article/S0165-1781(09)00161-9/abstract.

33. B. P. Hasler et al. "Phase Relationships between Core Body Temperature, Melatonin, and Sleep Are Associated with Depression Severity: Further Evidence for Circadian Misalignment in Non-Seasonal Depression." *Psychiatry Research* 178, no. 1 (2010): 205–207. http://www.psy-journal.com/article /S0165-1781(10)00186-1/fulltext.

34. T. Eckle. "Health Impact and Management of a Disrupted Circadian Rhythm and Sleep in Critical Illnesses." *Current Pharmaceutical Design* 21, no. 24 (2015): 3428–3430. https://www.ncbi.nlm.nih.gov/pmc/articles/PMC 4673005/#R9.

35. S. K. Davies et al. "Effect of Sleep Deprivation on the Human Metabolome." Proceedings of the National Academy of Sciences of the United States of America 111, no. 29 (2014): 10761–10766.

36. A. W. McHill et al. "Impact of Circadian Misalignment on Energy Metabolism during Simulated Nightshift Work." Proceedings of the National Academy of Sciences of the United States of America 111, no. 48 (2014): 17302–17307.

37. Ibid.

38. Ibid.

39. Ibid.

40. M. A. Grandner et al. "The Use of Technology at Night: Impact on Sleep and Health." *Journal of Clinical Sleep Medicine* 9, no. 12 (2013): 1301–1302. http://www.aasmnet.org/jcsm/ViewAbstract.aspx?pid=29250.

41. J. Schmerler. "Q&A: Why Is Blue Light before Bedtime Bad for Sleep?" *Scientific American.* September 1, 2015. https://www.scientificamerican.com /article/q-a-why-is-blue-light-before-bedtime-bad-for-sleep.

42. "International Tourist Arrivals Up 4% in the First Half of 2016." United Nations World Tourism Organization, September 29, 2016. Press release no. 16067. http://media.unwto.org/press-release/2016-09-26/international-tourist -arrivals-4-first-half-2016.

43. "What's Changed in Air Travel Since 1960?" International Association for Medical Assistance to Travelers, June 22, 2015. https://www.iamat .org/blog/whats-changed-in-air-travel-since-1960.

44. K. Cho et al. "Chronic Jet Lag Produces Cognitive Deficits." *Journal of Neuroscience* 20, no. RC66 (2000): 1–5. http://www.jneurosci.org/content /20/6/RC66.long.

45. E. Filipski et al. "Effects of Chronic Jet Lag on Tumor Progression in Mice." *Cancer Research* 64, no. 21 (2004): 7879–7885. https://www.ncbi .nlm.nih.gov/pubmed/15520194.

46. "Labor Movement." History Channel. http://www.history.com /topics/labor.

47. A. Sifferlin. "Working Too Hard? Physically Demanding Jobs Tied to Higher Risk of Heart Disease." *Time*. April 19, 2013. http://healthland .time.com/2013/04/19/physically-demanding-jobs-are-linked-to-higher -risk-of-heart-disease.

48. G. Reynolds. "Sit Less, Live Longer?" *The NYT Well Blog*, September 17, 2014. http://well.blogs.nytimes.com/2014/09/17/sit-less-live -longer/?_r=1.

49. N. Owen et al. "Sedentary Behavior: Emerging Evidence for a New Health Risk." *Mayo Clinic Proceedings* 85, no. 12 (2010): 1138–1141. https:// www.ncbi.nlm.nih.gov/pmc/articles/PMC2996155.

50. Ibid.

51. J. K. Goodrich et al. "Human Genetics Shape the Gut Micro-biome." *Cell* 159, no. 4 (2014): 789–799. https://www.ncbi.nlm.nih.gov /pubmed/25417156.

52. M. Chopra et al. "A Global Response to a Global Problem: The Epidemic of Overnutrition." *Bulletin of the World Health Organization* 80, no. 12 (2002). http://www.scielosp.org/scielo.php?script=sci_arttext&pid=S0042-9686200 2001200009.

Chapter 3: The Misinformation Highway

1. C. E. Kearns et al. "Sugar Industry and Coronary Heart Disease Research: A Historical Analysis of Internal Industry Documents." *JAMA Internal Medicine* 176, no. 11 (2016): 1680–1685. http://jamanetwork.com/journals/jamain ternalmedicine/article-abstract/2548255.

2. R. B. McGandy et al. "Dietary Fats, Carbohydrates and Atherosclerotic Vascular Disease." *New England Journal of Medicine* 3, no. 277: 245–247. https:// www.ncbi.nlm.nih.gov/pubmed/5339699.

3. A. O'Connor. "How the Sugar Industry Shifted Blame to Fat." *New York Times*, September 12, 2016. http://www.nytimes.com/2016/09/13/well/eat /how-the-sugar-industry-shifted-blame-to-fat.html?_r=1.

4. M. Nestle. "Food Lobbies, the Food Pyramid, and U.S. Nutrition Policy." *International Journal of Health Services* 23, no. 3 (1993): 483–496. https://www.ncbi.nlm.nih.gov/pubmed/8375951.

5. C. Choi. "AP Exclusive: How Candy Makers Shape Nutrition Science." *Associated Press*, June 2, 2016. http://bigstory.ap.org/article/f9483d554430445 fa6566bb0aaa293d1/ap-exclusive-how-candy-makers-shape-nutrition-science.

6. Ibid.

7. M. Nestle. "Six Industry-Funded Studies. The Score for the Year: 156/12." Food Politics, March 18, 2016. http://www.foodpolitics.com/2016/03/six -industry-funded-studies-the-score-for-the-year-15612.

8. A. Nevala-Lee. "Albert Einstein on Asking the Right Questions." *Wordpress*, June 2011. https://nevalalee.wordpress.com/2011/06/12/albert -einstein-on-asking-the-right-questions.

Chapter 4: Everything You Thought You Knew about Nutrition May Be Wrong

1. "The Food Guide Pyramid." United States Department of Agriculture, Center for Nutrition Policy and Promotion, October 1996. https://www .cnpp.usda.gov/sites/default/files/archived_projects/FGPPamphlet.pdf.

2. H. Antecol and K. Bedard. "Unhealthy Assimilation: Why Do Immigrants Converge to American Health Status Levels?" *Demography* 43, no. 2 (2006): 337–360. http://link.springer.com/article/10.1353/dem.2006.0011.

3. C. H. Barcenas et al. "Birthplace, Years of Residence in the United States, and Obesity among Mexican-American Adults." *Obesity* 15, no. 4 (2007): 1043–1052. http://onlinelibrary.wiley.com/doi/10.1038/oby.2007.537/full.

4. W. P. Frisbie et al. "Immigration and the Health of Asian and Pacific Islander Adults in the United States." *American Journal of Epidemiology* 153, no. 4 (2001): 372–380. https://www.ncbi.nlm.nih.gov/pubmed/11207155.

5. M. Sanghavi Goel et al. "Obesity among US Immigrant Subgroups by Duration of Residence." *JAMA* 292, no. 23 (2004): 2860–2867. http://jama network.com/journals/jama/fullarticle/199990.

6. R. D. Mattes and B. M. Popkin. "Nonnutritive Sweetener Consumption in Humans: Effects on Appetite and Food Intake and Their Putative Mechanisms." *American Journal of Clinical Nutrition* 89, no. 1 (2009): 1–14. http:// ajcn.nutrition.org/content/89/1/1.full.

7. J. Suez et al. "Artificial Sweeteners Induce Glucose Intolerance by Altering the Gut Microbiota." *Nature* 514, no. 7521 (2014): 181–186. http:// www.nature.com/nature/journal/v514/n7521/full/nature13793.html.

8. G. L. Austin et al. "Trends in Carbohydrate, Fat, and Protein Intakes and Association with Energy Intake in Normal-Weight, Overweight, and Obese Individuals: 1971–2006." *American Journal of Clinical Nutrition* 93, no. 4 (2011): 836–843. http://ajcn.nutrition.org/content/93/4/836.full.

9. V. L. Veum et al. "Visceral Adiposity and Metabolic Syndrome After Very High-Fat and Low-Fat Isocaloric Diets: A Randomized Controlled Trial." *American Journal of Clinical Nutrition*, November 30, 2016. http:// ajcn.nutrition.org/content/early/2016/11/30/ajcn.115.123463.abstract.

10. P. J. Turnbaugh et al. "An Obesity-Associated Gut Microbiome with Increased Capacity for Energy Harvest." *Nature* 444, no. 7122 (2006): 1027–1031. https://www.ncbi.nlm.nih.gov/pubmed/17183312.

11. "Majority of Studies of High-Fat Diets in Mice Inaccurately Portrayed." *UC Davis Health System.* http://www.ucdmc.ucdavis.edu/welcome/features/20080702_diet_warden.

12. C. Nierenberg. "Trans Fat Linked to Heart Disease, Huge Study Review Concludes." *Live Science*, August 11, 2015. http://www.livescience.com/51823-trans-fat-heart-disease.html.

13. M. U. Jakobsen et al. "Major Types of Dietary Fat and Risk of Coronary Heart Disease: A Pooled Analysis of 11 Cohort Studies." *American Journal of Clinical Nutrition* 89, no. 5 (2009): 1425–1432. https://www.ncbi.nlm.nih.gov/pmc/articles/PMC2676998.

14. M. U. Jakobsen et al. "Intake of Carbohydrates Compared with Intake of Saturated Fatty Acids and Risk of Myocardial Infarction: Importance of the Glycemic Index." *American Journal of Clinical Nutrition* 91, no. 6 (2010): 1764–1768. https://www.ncbi.nlm.nih.gov/pubmed/20375186.

15. R. Buettner et al. "Defining High-Fat-Diet Rat Models: Metabolic and Molecular Effects of Different Fat Types." *Journal of Molecular Endocrinology* 36, no. 3 (2006): 485–501. https://www.ncbi.nlm.nih.gov/pubmed/16720718.

16. R. J. de Souza et al. "Intake of Saturated and Trans Unsaturated Fatty Acids and Risk of All Cause Mortality, Cardiovascular Disease, and Type 2 Diabetes: Systematic Review and Meta-Analysis of Observational Studies." *British Medical Journal*, August 12, 2015. http://www.bmj.com/content/351/bmj.h3978.

17. L. A. Bazzano et al. "Effects of Low-Carbohydrate and Low-Fat Diets: A Randomized Trial." *Annals of Internal Medicine* 161, no. 5 (2014): 309–318. http://annals.org/aim/article/1900694/effects-low-carbohydrate-low-fat-diets-randomized-trial.

18. P. W. Siri-Tarino et al. "Meta-Analysis of Prospective Cohort Studies Evaluating the Association of Saturated Fat with Cardiovascular Disease." *American Journal of Clinical Nutrition*, January 13, 2010. http://ajcn.nutrition.org/content/early/2010/01/13/ajcn.2009.27725.abstract.

19. I. Shai et al. "Weight Loss with a Low-Carbohydrate, Mediterranean, or Low-Fat Diet." *New England Journal of Medicine* 359, no. 3 (2008): 229–241. https://www.ncbi.nlm.nih.gov/pubmed/18635428.

20. Nurses' Health Study. http://www.nurseshealthstudy.org.

21. Framingham Heart Study. https://www.framinghamheartstudy.org.

22. R. Chowdhury et al. "Association of Dietary, Circulating, and Supplement Fatty Acids with Coronary Risk: A Systematic Review and Meta-analysis."

Annals of Internal Medicine 160, no. 6 (2014): 398–406. http://annals.org /aim/article/1846638/association-dietary-circulating-supplement-fatty -acids-coronary-risk-systematic-review.

23. F. B. Hu et al. "Dietary Saturated Fats and Their Food Sources in Relation to the Risk of Coronary Heart Disease in Women." *American Journal of Clinical Nutrition* 70, no. 6 (1999): 1001–1008. https://www.ncbi.nlm.nih .gov/pubmed/10584044.

24. "The American Heart Association's Diet and Lifestyle Recommendations." *American Heart Association,* October 24, 2016. http://www.heart .org/HEARTORG/HealthyLiving/HealthyEating/Nutrition/The-American -Heart-Associations-Diet-and-Lifestyle-Recommendations_UCM_305855 _Article.jsp#.WEBp8eYrKUk.

25. L. R. Freeman et al. "Damaging Effects of a High-Fat Diet to the Brain and Cognition: A Review of Proposed Mechanisms." *Nutritional Neuroscience* 17, no. 6 (2014): 241–251. https://www.ncbi.nlm.nih.gov/pmc/articles /PMC4074256.

26. S. Kalmijn et al. "Dietary Fat Intake and the Risk of Incident Dementia in the Rotterdam Study." *Annals of Neurology* 42, no. 5 (1997): 776–782. https://www.ncbi.nlm.nih.gov/pubmed/9392577.

27. A. H. Lichtenstein and L. Van Horn. "Very Low Fat Diets." *Circulation* 8, no. 9 (1998): 935–939. http://circ.ahajournals.org/content/98/9/935.

28. N. A. Graudal et al. "Effects of Sodium Restriction on Blood Pressure, Renin, Aldosterone, Catecholamines, Cholesterols, and Triglyceride: A Meta-analysis." *JAMA* 279, no. 17 (1998): 1383–1391. http://jamanetwork.com /journals/jama/article-abstract/187486.

29. S. J. Ley et al. "Long-Term Effects of a Reduced Fat Diet Intervention on Cardiovascular Disease Risk Factors in Individuals with Glucose Intolerance." *Diabetes Research and Clinical Practice* 63, no. 2 (2004): 103–112. http://www .diabetesresearchclinicalpractice.com/article/S0168-8227(03)00218-3/abstract.

30. N. Mansoor et al. "Effects of Low-Carbohydrate Diets v. Low-Fat Diets on Body Weight and Cardiovascular Risk Factors: A Meta-analysis of Randomized Controlled Trials." *British Journal of Nutrition* 115, no. 3 (2016): 466–479. https://www.ncbi.nlm.nih.gov/pubmed/26768850.

31. S. J. Ley et al. "Long-Term Effects of a Reduced Fat Diet Intervention on Cardiovascular Disease Risk Factors in Individuals with Glucose Intolerance." *Diabetes Research and Clinical Practice* 63, no. 2 (2004): 103–112. http:// www.diabetesresearchclinicalpractice.com/article/S0168-8227(03)00218-3 /abstract.

32. Ibid.

33. A. H. Lichtenstein and L. Van Horn. "Very Low Fat Diets." *Circulation* 98, no. 9 (1998): 935–939. http://circ.ahajournals.org/content/98/9/935.

34. E. J. Schaefer et al. "The Effects of Low Cholesterol, High Polyunsaturated Fat, and Low Fat Diets on Plasma Lipid and Lipoprotein Cholesterol Levels in Normal and Hypercholesterolemic Subjects." *American Journal of Clinical Nutrition* 34, no. 9 (1981): 1758–1763. http://ajcn.nutrition.org/content/34/9/1758?ijkey=f83315783c84ba9ee2a161b04e572d5d2925add0&keytype2=tf_ipsecsha.

35. J. M. Lattimer and M. D. Haub. "Effects of Dietary Fiber and Its Components on Metabolic Health." *Nutrients* 2, no. 12 (2010): 1266–1289. https://www.ncbi.nlm.nih.gov/pmc/articles/PMC3257631.

36. Q. Yang et al. "Added Sugar Intake and Cardiovascular Diseases Mortality among US Adults." *JAMA Internal Medicine* 174, no. 4 (2014): 516–524. http://jamanetwork.com/journals/jamainternalmedicine/fullarticle/1819573.

37. L. S. Gross et al. "Increased Consumption of Refined Carbohydrates and the Epidemic of Type 2 Diabetes in the United States: An Ecologic Assessment." *American Journal of Clinical Nutrition* 79, no. 5 (2004): 774–779. http://ajcn.nutrition.org/content/79/5/774.full.

38. S. S. Jonnalagadda et al. "Putting the Whole Grain Puzzle Together: Health Benefits Associated with Whole Grains—Summary of American Society for Nutrition 2010 Satellite Symposium." *Journal of Nutrition* 141, no. 5 (2011): 1011S–1022S. https://www.ncbi.nlm.nih.gov/pmc/articles/PMC3078018.

39. Q. Yang et al. "Added Sugar Intake and Cardiovascular Diseases Mortality among US Adults." *Jama Internal Medicine* 174, no. 4 (2014): 516–524. http://jamanetwork.com/journals/jamainternalmedicine/fullarticle/1819573.

40. L. R. Vartanian et al. "Effects of Soft Drink Consumption on Nutrition and Health: A Systematic Review and Meta-analysis." *American Journal of Public Health* 97, no. 4 (2007): 667–675. https://www.ncbi.nlm.nih.gov/pmc/articles/PMC1829363.

41. L. S. Gross et al. "Increased Consumption of Refined Carbohydrates and the Epidemic of Type 2 Diabetes in the United States: An Ecologic Assessment." *American Journal of Clinical Nutrition* 79, no. 5 (2004): 774–779. http://ajcn.nutrition.org/content/79/5/774.full.

42. S. Apple. "An Old Idea, Revived: Starve Cancer to Death." *New York Times Magazine*, May 12, 2016. http://www.nytimes.com/2016/05/15/magazine/warburg-effect-an-old-idea-revived-starve-cancer-to-death.html?_r=2.

43. "The Framingham Diet Study: Diet and the Regulation of Serum Cholesterol." U.S. Department of Health, Education, and Welfare, Public Health

Service, National Institutes of Health, 1971. https://books.google.com.au /books/about/The_Framingham_diet_study.html?id=-JzIHAAACAAJ.

44. E. Fothergill et al. "Persistent Metabolic Adaptation 6 Years after 'The Biggest Loser' Competition." *Obesity* 24, no. 8 (2016): 1612–1619. http:// onlinelibrary.wiley.com/doi/10.1002/oby.21538/full#oby21538-bib-0038.

45. K. H. Pietiläinen et al. "Does Dieting Make You Fat? A Twin Study." *International Journal of Obesity* 36 (2012): 456–464. http://www.nature .com/ijo/journal/v36/n3/full/ijo2011160a.html.

46. A. E. Field et al. "Relation Between Dieting and Weight Change Among Preadolescents and Adolescents." *Pediatrics* 112, no. 4 (2003). http:// pediatrics.aappublications.org/content/112/4/900.

47. D. Neumark-Sztainer et al. "Obesity, Disordered Eating, and Eating Disorders in a Longitudinal Study of Adolescents: How Do Dieters Fare 5 Years Later?" *Journal of the American Dietetic Association* 106, no. 4 (2006): 559–568. https://www.ncbi.nlm.nih.gov/pubmed/16567152.

48. G. C. Patton et al. "Onset of Adolescent Eating Disorders: Population Based Cohort Study over 3 Years." *British Medical Journal* 318 (1999): 765. http://www.bmj.com/content/318/7186/765?view=long&pmid=10082698.

Chapter 5: The Universe Inside Your Gut—And Why It Matters

1. F. Marineli et al. "Mary Mallon (1869–1938) and the History of Typhoid Fever." *Annals of Gastroenterology* 26, no. 2 (2013): 132–134. https://www.ncbi.nlm.nih.gov/pmc/articles/PMC3959940/pdf/AnnGastro enterol-26-132.pdf.

2. "Typhoid Fever." WebMD. http://www.webmd.com/a-to-z-guides /typhoid-fever#1.

3. T. Hesman Saey. "Body's Bacteria Don't Outnumber Human Cells So Much after All." *Science News*, January 8, 2016. https://www.sciencenews .org/article/body%E2%80%99s-bacteria-don%E2%80%99t-outnumber -human-cells-so-much-after-all.

4. Ibid.

5. J. Debelius et al. "Tiny Microbes, Enormous Impacts: What Matters in Gut Microbiome Studies?" *Genome Biology*, October 19, 2016. http://genome biology.biomedcentral.com/articles/10.1186/s13059-016-1086-x#CR1.

6. "Fast Facts about the Human Microbiome." Center for Ecogenetics & Environmental Health, January 2014. https://depts.washington.edu/ceeh /downloads/FF_Microbiome.pdf.

7. P. J. Turnbaugh et al. "An Obesity-Associated Gut Microbiome with Increased Capacity for Energy Harvest." *Nature* 444 (2006): 1027–1031.

http://www.nature.com/nature/journal/v444/n7122/abs/nature05414
.html.

8. Ibid.

9. "Beneficial Gut Bacteria That Produce Vitamins B2, B9, B12 and K2." *Eupedia*, February 14, 2016. http://www.eupedia.com/forum/threads/31972 -Beneficial-gut-bacteria-that-produce-vitamins-B2-B9-B12-and-K2.

10. Ibid.

11. Ibid.

12. "The Human Microbiome, Diet, and Health: Workshop Summary." Institute of Medicine, Health and Medicine Division, 2013. https://www .ncbi.nlm.nih.gov/books/NBK154098.

13. "Microbiome 101: Understanding Gut Microbiota." Prescript-Assist. http://www.prescript-assist.com/intestinal-health/gut-microbiome.

14. V. K. Ridaura et al. "Gut Microbiota from Twins Discordant for Obesity Modulate Metabolism in Mice." *Science* 341, no. 6150 (2013). http:// science.sciencemag.org/content/341/6150/1241214.

15. J. K. Goodrich et al. "Human Genetics Shape the Gut Microbiome." *Cell* 159, no. 4 (2014): 789–799. http://www.cell.com/cell/fulltext/S0092 -8674(14)01241-0.

16. M. Noval Rivas et al. "A Microbiota Signature Associated with Experimental Food Allergy Promotes Allergic Sensitization and Anaphylaxis." *Journal of Allergy and Clinical Immunology* 131, no. 1 (2013): 201–212. http:// www.jacionline.org/article/S0091-6749(12)01694-6/abstract.

17. A. D. Kostic et al. "The Dynamics of the Human Infant Gut Microbiome in Development and in Progression toward Type 1 Diabetes." *Cell Host & Microbiome* 17, no. 2 (2015): 260–273. http://www.cell.com/cell-host-microbe /fulltext/S1931-3128(16)30264-5.

18. X. Zhang et al. "The Oral and Gut Microbiomes Are Perturbed in Rheumatoid Arthritis and Partly Normalized after Treatment." *Nature Medicine* 21 (2015): 895–905. http://www.nature.com/nm/journal/v21/n8/full /nm.3914.html.

19. M. E. Costello et al. "Brief Report: Intestinal Dysbiosis in Ankylosing Spondylitis." *Arthritis & Rheumatology* 67, no. 3 (2015): 686–691. http:// onlinelibrary.wiley.com/doi/10.1002/art.38967/abstract.

20. M. C. de Goffau et al. "Fecal Microbiota Composition Differs between Children with β-Cell Autoimmunity and Those Without." *Diabetes* 62, no. 4 (2013): 1238–1244. http://diabetes.diabetesjournals.org/content /62/4/1238.

21. A. Giongo et al. "Toward Defining the Autoimmune Microbiome for Type 1 Diabetes." *ISME Journal* 5 (2011): 82–91. http://www.nature.com /ismej/journal/v5/n1/full/ismej201092a.html.

22. S. Michail et al. "Alterations in the Gut Microbiome of Children with Severe Ulcerative Colitis." *Inflammatory Bowel Diseases* 18, no. 10 (2012): 1799–1808. https://www.ncbi.nlm.nih.gov/pubmed/22170749.

23. R. A. Luna and J. A. Foster. "Gut Brain Axis: Diet Microbiota Interactions and Implications for Modulation of Anxiety and Depression." *Current Opinion in Biotechnology* 32 (2015): 35–41. https://www.ncbi.nlm.nih.gov/pubmed/25448230.

24. S. Dash et al. "The Gut Microbiome and Diet in Psychiatry: Focus on Depression." *Current Opinion in Psychiatry* 28, no. 1 (2015): 1–6. https://www.ncbi.nlm.nih.gov/pubmed/25415497.

25. S. C. Kleinman et al. "The Intestinal Microbiota in Acute Anorexia Nervosa and During Renourishment: Relationship to Depression, Anxiety, and Eating Disorder Psychopathology." *Psychosomatic Medicine* 77, no. 9 (2015): 969–981. https://www.ncbi.nlm.nih.gov/pubmed/26428446.

26. E. Castro-Nallar et al. "Composition, Taxonomy and Functional Diversity of the Oropharynx Microbiome in Individuals with Schizophrenia and Controls." *PeerJ*, August 2015. https://peerj.com/articles/1140.

27. A. Keshavarzian et al. "Colonic Bacterial Composition in Parkinson's Disease." *Movement Disorders* 30, no. 10 (2015): 1351–1360. http://onlinelibrary.wiley.com/doi/10.1002/mds.26307/abstract.

28. J. M. Hill et al. "Pathogenic Microbes, the Microbiome, and Alzheimer's Disease (AD)." *Frontiers in Aging Neuroscience* 6 (2014): 127. https://www.ncbi.nlm.nih.gov/pmc/articles/PMC4058571.

29. Y. Zhao and W. J. Lukiw. "Microbiome-Generated Amyloid and Potential Impact on Amyloidogenesis in Alzheimer's Disease (AD)." *Journal of Nature and Science* 1, no. 7 (2015). https://www.ncbi.nlm.nih.gov/pubmed/26097896.

30. Z. Wang et al. "Gut Flora Metabolism of Phosphatidylcholine Promotes Cardiovascular Disease." *Nature* 472, no. 7341 (2011): 57–63. http://www.nature.com/nature/journal/v472/n7341/full/nature09922.html.

31. W. Tang et al. "Intestinal Microbial Metabolism of Phosphatidylcholine and Cardiovascular Risk." *New England Journal of Medicine* 368 (2013): 1575–1584. http://www.nejm.org/doi/full/10.1056/NEJMoa1109400.

32. N. T. Mueller et al. "The Infant Microbiome Development: Mom Matters." *Trends in Molecular Medicine* 21, no. 2 (2015): 109–117. https://www.ncbi.nlm.nih.gov/pmc/articles/PMC4464665.

33. P. W. O'Toole and I. B. Jeffery. "Gut Microbiota and Aging." *Science* 350, no. 6265 (2015): 1214–1215. https://www.ncbi.nlm.nih.gov/pubmed/26785481.

34. E. D. Sonnenburg et al. "Diet-Induced Extinctions in the Gut Microbiota Compound over Generations." *Nature* 529, no. 7585 (2016): 212–215. http://www.nature.com/nature/journal/v529/n7585/full/nature16504.html.

35. "Low-Fiber Diet May Cause Irreversible Depletion of Gut Bacteria over Generations." *Stanford University Medical Center*, January 13, 2016. https://www.sciencedaily.com/releases/2016/01/160113160657.htm.

36. R. J. Perry et al. "Acetate Mediates a Microbiome-Brain-β-Cell Axis to Promote Metabolic Syndrome." *Nature* 534, no. 7606 (2016): 213–217. https://www.ncbi.nlm.nih.gov/pubmed/27279214.

37. F. De Vadder et al. "Microbiota-Produced Succinate Improves Glucose Homeostasis via Intestinal Gluconeogenesis." *Cell Metabolism* 24, no. 1 (2016): 151–157. https://www.ncbi.nlm.nih.gov/pubmed/27411015.

38. A. Vrieze et al. "Transfer of Intestinal Microbiota from Lean Donors Increases Insulin Sensitivity in Individuals with Metabolic Syndrome." *Gastroenterology* 143, no. 4 (2012): 913–916. http://www.gastrojournal.org/article/S0016-5085(12)00892-X/abstract.

39. R. A. Koeth et al. "Intestinal Microbiota Metabolism of L-carnitine, a Nutrient in Red Meat, Promotes Atherosclerosis." *Nature Medicine* 19 (2013): 576–585. http://www.nature.com/nm/journal/v19/n5/full/nm.3145.html.

40. C. Woolston. "Red Meat + Wrong Bacteria = Bad News for Hearts." *Nature*, April 7, 2013. http://www.nature.com/news/red-meat-wrong-bacteria-bad-news-for-hearts-1.12746.

41. "Researchers Find New Link between Red Meat and Heart Disease." *Cleveland Clinic*, November 11, 2014. https://health.clevelandclinic.org/2014/11/researchers-find-new-link-between-red-meat-and-heart-disease-video.

42. "Fast Facts about the Human Microbiome." Center for Ecogenetics & Environmental Health, January 2014. https://depts.washington.edu/ceeh/downloads/FF_Microbiome.pdf.

43. P. J. Turnbaugh et al. "An Obesity-Associated Gut Microbiome with Increased Capacity for Energy Harvest." *Nature* 444 (2006): 1027–1031. http://www.nature.com/nature/journal/v444/n7122/abs/nature05414.html.

44. V. K. Ridaura et al. "Cultured Gut Microbiota from Twins Discordant for Obesity Modulate Adiposity and Metabolic Phenotypes in Mice." *Science* 341, no. 6150 (2013). https://www.ncbi.nlm.nih.gov/pmc/articles/PMC3829625.

45. C. A. Thaiss et al. "Persistent Microbiome Alterations Modulate the Rate of Post-Dieting Weight Regain." *Nature* 540, no. 7634 (2016): 544–551. http://www.nature.com/nature/journal/v540/n7634/full/nature20796.html.

46. R. E. Ley et al. "Worlds within Worlds: Evolution of the Vertebrate Gut Microbiota." *Nature Reviews Microbiology* 6 (2008): 776–788. http://www.nature.com/nrmicro/journal/v6/n10/full/nrmicro1978.html.

47. F. Godoy-Vitorino et al. "Comparative Analyses of Foregut and Hindgut Bacterial Communities in Hoatzins and Cows." *ISME Journal* 6 (2012): 531–541. http://www.nature.com/ismej/journal/v6/n3/full/ismej2011131a.html.

48. J. G. Sanders et al. "Baleen Whales Host a Unique Gut Microbiome with Similarities to Both Carnivores and Herbivores." *Nature* 6, no. 8285 (2015). http://www.nature.com/articles/ncomms9285.

49. L. Zhu et al. "Evidence of Cellulose Metabolism by the Giant Panda Gut Microbiome." *PNAS* 108, no. 43 (2011): 17714–17719. http://www.pnas.org/content/108/43/17714.

50. T. Yatsunenko et al. "Human Gut Microbiome Viewed across Age and Geography." *Nature* 486, no. 7402 (2012): 222–227. http://www.nature.com/nature/journal/v486/n7402/full/nature11053.html.

51. J. E. Koenig et al. "Succession of Microbial Consortia in the Developing Infant Gut Microbiome." *PNAS* 108 (2010). http://www.pnas.org/content/108/Supplement_1/4578.

52. F. Bäckhed et al. "Dynamics and Stabilization of the Human Gut Microbiome during the First Year of Life." *Cell Host & Microbe* 17, no. 5 (2015): 852. http://www.cell.com/cell-host-microbe/fulltext/S1931-3128(15)00216-4.

53. T. Yatsunenko et al. "Human Gut Microbiome Viewed across Age and Geography." *Nature* 486, no. 7402 (2012): 222–227. http://www.nature.com/nature/journal/v486/n7402/full/nature11053.html.

54. J. C. Clemente et al. "The Microbiome of Uncontacted Amerindians." *Science Advances* 1, no. 3 (2015). http://advances.sciencemag.org/content/1/3/e1500183.

55. I. Cho et al. "Antibiotics in Early Life Alter the Murine Colonic Microbiome and Adiposity." *Nature* 488, no. 7413 (2012): 621–626. http://www.nature.com/nature/journal/v488/n7413/full/nature11400.html.

56. K. Korpela et al. "Intestinal Microbiome Is Related to Lifetime Antibiotic Use in Finnish Pre-School Children." *Nature Communications* 7, no. 10410 (2016). http://www.nature.com/articles/ncomms10410.

57. H. E. Jakobsson et al. "Short-Term Antibiotic Treatment Has Differing Long-Term Impacts on the Human Throat and Gut Microbiome." *PLoS One* 5, no. 3 (2010). http://journals.plos.org/plosone/article?id=10.1371/journal.pone.0009836.

58. L. Dethlefsen and D. A. Relman. "Incomplete Recovery and Individualized Responses of the Human Distal Gut Microbiota to Repeated Antibiotic Perturbation." *PNAS*, August 17, 2010. http://www.pnas.org/content/108/Supplement_1/4554.

59. G. D. Wu et al. "Linking Long-Term Dietary Patterns with Gut Microbial Enterotypes." *Science* 334, no. 6052 (2011): 105–108. http://science.sciencemag.org/content/334/6052/105.

60. E. D. Sonnenburg et al. "Diet-Induced Extinctions in the Gut Microbiota Compound over Generations." *Nature* 529, no. 7585 (2016): 212–215. http://www.nature.com/nature/journal/v529/n7585/full/nature16504.html.

61. C. F. Maurice et al. "Xenobiotics Shape the Physiology and Gene Expression of the Active Human Gut Microbiome." *Cell* 152, nos. 1–2 (2013): 39–50. http://www.cell.com/cell/fulltext/S0092-8674(12)01428-6.

62. M. A. Jackson et al. "Proton Pump Inhibitors Alter the Composition of the Gut Microbiota." *Gut* 65, no. 5 (2015): 749–756. http://gut.bmj.com/content/65/5/749.

63. D. E. Freedberg et al. "Proton Pump Inhibitors Alter Specific Taxa in the Human Gastrointestinal Microbiome: A Crossover Trial." *Gastroenterology* 149, no. 4 (2015): 883–885. http://www.gastrojournal.org/article/S0016-5085(15)00933-6/fulltext.

64. K. Forslund et al. "Disentangling Type 2 Diabetes and Metformin Treatment Signatures in the Human Gut Microbiota." *Nature* 528, no. 7581 (2015): 262–266. http://www.nature.com/nature/journal/v528/n7581/full/nature15766.html.

65. M. G. Rooks et al. "Gut Microbiome Composition and Function in Experimental Colitis during Active Disease and Treatment-Induced Remission." *ISME Journal* 8 (2014): 1403–1417. http://www.nature.com/ismej/journal/v8/n7/full/ismej20143a.html.

66. E. Mendes. "Personalized Cancer Care: Where It Stands Today." American Cancer Society (2015). https://www.cancer.org/latest-news/personalized-cancer-care-where-it-stands-today.html.

67. J. K. Goodrich et al. "Human Genetics Shape the Gut Microbiome." *Cell* 159, no. 4 (2014): 789–799. http://www.cell.com/cell/fulltext/S0092-8674(14)01241-0.

68. P. J. Turnbaugh et al. "A Core Gut Microbiome in Obese and Lean Twins." *Nature* 457 (2009): 480–484. http://www.nature.com/nature/journal/v457/n7228/full/nature07540.html.

69. N. Kodaman et al. "Human and *Helicobacter pylori* Coevolution Shapes the Risk of Gastric Disease." *PNAS* 111, no. 4 (2013): 1455–1460. http://www.pnas.org/content/111/4/1455.

70. S. S. Kang et al. "Diet and Exercise Orthogonally Alter the Gut Microbiome and Reveal Independent Associations with Anxiety and Cognition." *Molecular Neurodegeneration* 9, no. 36 (2014). http://molecularneurodegeneration.biomedcentral.com/articles/10.1186/1750-1326-9-36.

71. S. F. Clarke et al. "Exercise and Associated Dietary Extremes Impact on Gut Microbial Diversity." *Gut* 63, no. 12 (2014): 1913–1920. http://gut.bmj.com/content/63/12/1913.

72. J. E. Lambert et al. "Exercise Training Modifies Gut Microbiota in Normal and Diabetic Mice." *Applied Physiology, Nutrition, and Metabolism* 40, no. 7 (2015): 749–752. http://www.nrcresearchpress.com/doi/abs/10.1139/apnm-2014-0452#.WEL9tfkrLIU.

73. S. J. Song et al. "Cohabiting Family Members Share Microbiota with One Another and with Their Dogs." *eLife*, April 16, 2013. https://elifesciences.org/content/2/e00458.

74. G. D. Wu et al. "Linking Long-Term Dietary Patterns with Gut Microbial Enterotypes." *Science* 334, no. 6052 (2011): 105–108. http://science.sciencemag.org/content/334/6052/105.

75. L. A. David et al. "Diet Rapidly and Reproducibly Alters the Human Gut Microbiome." *Nature* 505, no. 7484 (2014): 559–563. http://www.nature.com/nature/journal/v505/n7484/full/nature12820.html.

76. C. A. Thaiss et al. "Transkingdom Control of Microbiota Diurnal Oscillations Promotes Metabolic Homeostasis." *Cell* 159, no. 3 (2014): 514–529. http://www.cell.com/abstract/S0092-8674(14)01236-7.

77. A. Park. "Why Shift Work and Sleeplessness Lead to Weight Gain and Diabetes." *Time*, April 12, 2012. http://healthland.time.com/2012/04/12/why-shift-work-and-sleeplessness-lead-to-weight-gain-and-diabetes.

78. L. Blue. "It's Called the Graveyard Shift for a Reason." *Time*, July 27, 2012. http://healthland.time.com/2012/07/27/its-called-the-graveyard-shift-for-a-reason.

79. A. Park. "Working the Night Shift May Boost Breast Cancer Risk." *Time*, May 29, 2012. http://healthland.time.com/2012/05/29/working-the-night-shift-may-boost-breast-cancer-risk.

80. A. Park. "Why Working the Night Shift May Boost Your Risk of Diabetes." *Time*, December 7, 2011. http://healthland.time.com/2011/12/07/why-working-the-night-shift-may-boost-your-risk-of-diabetes.

81. C. A. Thaiss et al. "Transkingdom Control of Microbiota Diurnal Oscillations Promotes Metabolic Homeostasis." *Cell* 159, no. 3 (2014): 514–529. http://www.cell.com/abstract/S0092-8674(14)01236-7.

82. Ibid.

83. J. Suez et al. "Artificial Sweeteners Induce Glucose Intolerance by Altering the Gut Microbiota." *Nature* 514, no. 7521 (2014): 181–186. http://www.nature.com/nature/journal/v514/n7521/full/nature13793.html.

84. "Non-nutritive Sweeteners: A Potentially Useful Option—with Caveats." *American Heart Association, American Diabetes Association*, July 9, 2012. http://www.diabetes.org/newsroom/press-releases/2012/ada-aha-sweetener-statement.html.

Chapter 6: Blood Sugar: Your Ultimate Food Feedback Response

1. "What Is Diabetes?" Texas Diabetes Council. http://www.preventtype2.org/what-is-diabetes.php.

2. A. Gastaldelli et al. "Beta-Cell Dysfunction and Glucose Intolerance: Results from the San Antonio Metabolism (SAM) Study." *Diabetologia* 47, no. 1 (2004): 31–39. http://link.springer.com/article/10.1007/s00125-003-1263-9?LI=true.

3. A. E. Butler et al. "β-Cell Deficit and Increased β-Cell Apoptosis in Humans with Type 2 Diabetes." *Diabetes* 52, no. 1 (2003): 102–110. http://diabetes.diabetesjournals.org/content/52/1/102.full.

4. A. G. Tabák et al. "Prediabetes: A High-Risk State for Developing Diabetes." *Lancet* 379, no. 9833 (2012): 2279–2290. https://www.ncbi.nlm.nih.gov/pmc/articles/PMC3891203.

5. E. Selvin et al. "Glycemic Control and Coronary Heart Disease Risk in Persons with and without Diabetes: The Atherosclerosis Risk in Communities Study." *Archives of Internal Medicine* 165, no. 16 (2005): 1910–1916. https://www.ncbi.nlm.nih.gov/pubmed/16157837?dopt=Abstract.

6. K. T. Khaw et al. "Association of Hemoglobin A1c with Cardiovascular Disease and Mortality in Adults: The European Prospective Investigation into Cancer in Norfolk." *Annals of Internal Medicine* 141, no. 6 (2004): 413–420. https://www.ncbi.nlm.nih.gov/pubmed/15381514.

7. "Blood Sugar 101: What They Don't Tell You about Diabetes." http://www.phlaunt.com/diabetes/14046669.php.

8. L. Monnier et al. "Activation of Oxidative Stress by Acute Glucose Fluctuations Compared with Sustained Chronic Hyperglycemia in Patients with Type 2 Diabetes." *JAMA* 295, no. 14 (2006): 1681–1687. https://www.ncbi.nlm.nih.gov/pubmed/16609090.

9. "Research Connecting Organ Damage with Blood Sugar Level." *Blood Sugar 101.* http://www.phlaunt.com/diabetes/14045678.php.

10. B. Kaur et al. "The Impact of a Low Glycaemic Index (GI) Diet on Simultaneous Measurements of Blood Glucose and Fat Oxidation: A Whole Body Calorimetric Study." *Journal of Clinical & Translational Endocrinology* 4 (2016): 45–52. http://www.sciencedirect.com/science/article/pii/S2214623716300060.

11. D. B. Pawlak et al. "Effects of Dietary Glycaemic Index on Adiposity, Glucose Homeostasis, and Plasma Lipids in Animals." *Lancet* 364, no. 9436 (2004): 778–785. https://www.ncbi.nlm.nih.gov/pubmed/15337404.

12. N. Torbay et al. "Insulin Increases Body Fat Despite Control of Food Intake and Physical Activity." *American Journal of Physiology* 248, no. 1 pt. 2 (1985): R120–R124. https://www.ncbi.nlm.nih.gov/pubmed/3881983.

13. M. Bergman et al. "One-Hour Post-Load Plasma Glucose Level during the OGTT Predicts Mortality: Observations from the Israel Study of Glucose Intolerance, Obesity and Hypertension." *Diabetic Medicine* 33, no. 8 (2016): 1060–1066. http://onlinelibrary.wiley.com/doi/10.1111/dme.13116/abstract.

14. F. Cavalot et al. "Postprandial Blood Glucose Predicts Cardiovascular Events and All-Cause Mortality in Type 2 Diabetes in a 14-Year Follow-Up." *Diabetes Care* 34, no. 10 (2011): 2237–2243. http://care.diabetesjournals .org/content/34/10/2237.

15. G. Bardini et al. "Inflammation Markers and Metabolic Characteristics of Subjects with One-Hour Plasma Glucose Levels." *Diabetes Care*, November 2009. http://care.diabetesjournals.org/content/early/2009/11/12/dc09-1342.abstract.

16. T. S. Temelkova-Kurktschiev et al. "Postchallenge Plasma Glucose and Glycemic Spikes Are More Strongly Associated with Atherosclerosis Than Fasting Glucose or HbA1c Level." *Diabetes Care* 23, no. 12 (2000): 1830–1834. https://www.ncbi.nlm.nih.gov/pubmed/11128361.

17. N. Rabbani et al. "Glycation of LDL by Methylglyoxal Increases Arterial Atherogenicity." *Diabetes* 60, no. 7 (2011): 1973–1980. http://diabetes .diabetesjournals.org/content/60/7/1973.

18. "Research Connecting Organ Damage with Blood Sugar Level." *Blood Sugar 101*. http://www.phlaunt.com/diabetes/14045678.php.

19. S. Apple. "An Old Idea, Revived: Starve Cancer to Death." *New York Times Magazine*, May 12, 2016. http://www.nytimes.com/2016/05/15/magazine /warburg-effect-an-old-idea-revived-starve-cancer-to-death.html?_r=2.

20. "Research Connecting Organ Damage with Blood Sugar Level." *Blood Sugar 101*. http://www.phlaunt.com/diabetes/14045678.php.

21. P. Stattin et al. "Prospective Study of Hyperglycemia and Cancer Risk." *Diabetes Care* 30, no. 3 (2007): 561–567. https://www.ncbi.nlm.nih .gov/pubmed/17327321.

22. M. Davies. "'Quitting Carbs Has Saved My Life': Cancer Victim Given Months to Live Refuses Chemo and Claims Diet of Meat and Dairy Is Why He's Still Alive Two Years Later." *Daily Mail*, July 15, 2016. http://www .dailymail.co.uk/health/article-3691808/Quitting-carbs-saved-life-Cancer -victim-given-months-live-refuses-chemo-claims-diet-meat-dairy-s-alive -two-years-later.html.

23. V. W. Ho et al. "A Low Carbohydrate, High Protein Diet Slows Tumor Growth and Prevents Cancer Initiation." *Cancer Research* 71, no. 13 (2011): 4484–4493. http://cancerres.aacrjournals.org/content/early/2011/06/10/0008 -5472.CAN-10-3973.

24. University of Texas MD Anderson Cancer Center. "Sugars in Western Diets Increase Risk for Breast Cancer Tumors and Metastasis." January 4, 2016. https://www.sciencedaily.com/releases/2016/01/160104080034.htm.

25. Y. Jiang, et al. "Abstract 3735: Dietary Sugar Induces Tumorigenesis in Mammary Gland Partially through 12 Lipoxygenase Pathway." *Cancer Research* 75, no. 15, Supplement. http://cancerres.aacrjournals.org /content/75/15_Supplement/3735.

26. W. Q. Zhao et al. "Insulin Resistance and Amyloidogenesis as Common Molecular Foundation for Type 2 Diabetes and Alzheimer's Disease." *BBA Molecular Basis of Disease* 1792, no. 5 (2009): 482–496. http://www.sciencedirect.com/science/article/pii/S0925443908002093.

27. Ibid.

28. P. K. Crane et al. "Glucose Levels and Risk of Dementia." *New England Journal of Medicine* 369 (2013): 540–548. http://www.nejm.org/doi/full/10.1056/NEJMoa1215740.

29. N. Cherbuin. "Higher Normal Fasting Plasma Glucose Is Associated with Hippocampal Atrophy." *Neurology* 79, no. 10 (2012): 1019–1026. http://www.neurology.org/content/79/10/1019.

30. J. Robinson Singleton et al. "Increased Prevalence of Impaired Glucose Tolerance in Patients with Painful Sensory Neuropathy." *Diabetes Care* 24, no. 8 (2001): 1448–1453. http://care.diabetesjournals.org/content/24/8/1448.full.

31. C. J. Sumner et al. "The Spectrum of Neuropathy in Diabetes and Impaired Glucose Tolerance." *Neurology* 60, no. 1 (2003): 108–111. http://www.neurology.org/content/60/1/108.abstract.

32. O. P. Adams. "The Impact of Brief High-Intensity Exercise on Blood Glucose Levels." *Diabetes, Metabolic Syndrome and Obesity: Targets and Therapy* 6 (2013): 113–122. https://www.ncbi.nlm.nih.gov/pmc/articles/PMC3587394.

33. S. R. Colberg et al. "Blood Glucose Responses to Type, Intensity, Duration, and Timing of Exercise." *Diabetes Care* 36, no. 10 (2013): e177. http://care.diabetesjournals.org/content/36/10/e177.

34. M. C. Gannon and F. Q. Nuttall. "Effect of a High-Protein, Low-Carbohydrate Diet on Blood Glucose Control in People with Type 2 Diabetes." *Diabetes* 53, no. 9 (2004): 2375–2382. http://diabetes.diabetesjournals.org/content/53/9/2375.

35. R. D. Feinman et al. "Dietary Carbohydrate Restriction as the First Approach in Diabetes Management: Critical Review and Evidence Base." *Nutrition* 31, no. 1 (2015): 1–13. http://www.sciencedirect.com/science/article/pii/S0899900714003323.

36. E. J. Mayer-Davis. "Low-Fat Diets for Diabetes Prevention." *Diabetes Care* 24, no. 4 (2001): 613–614. http://care.diabetesjournals.org/content/24/4/613.

37. N. D. Barnard et al. "A Low-Fat Vegan Diet Improves Glycemic Control and Cardiovascular Risk Factors in a Randomized Clinical Trial in Individuals with Type 2 Diabetes." *Diabetes Care* 29, no. 8 (2006): 1777–1783. http://care.diabetesjournals.org/content/29/8/1777.

38. J. S. de Munter et al. "Whole Grain, Bran, and Germ Intake and Risk of Type 2 Diabetes: A Prospective Cohort Study and Systematic Review." *PLoS Medicine* 4, no. 8 (2007): e261. https://www.ncbi.nlm.nih.gov/pubmed/17760498.

39. "Glycemic Index and Diabetes." *American Diabetes Association*, October 2, 2013. http://www.diabetes.org/food-and-fitness/food/what-can-i-eat/understanding-carbohydrates/glycemic-index-and-diabetes.html.

40. G. Radulian et al. "Metabolic Effects of Low Glycaemic Index Diets." *Nutrition Journal* 8, no. 5 (2009). https://www.ncbi.nlm.nih.gov/pmc/articles/PMC2654909.

41. "Healthy Eaters: Ignore Glycemic Index. Clinical Trial Shows No Beneficial Effects on Key Measures of Heart Disease and Diabetes Risk." *Johns Hopkins Medicine*, December 16, 2014.

42. K. L. Knutson. "Impact of Sleep and Sleep Loss on Glucose Homeostasis and Appetite Regulation." *Sleep Medicine Clinic* 2, no. 2 (2007): 187–197. https://www.ncbi.nlm.nih.gov/pmc/articles/PMC2084401.

43. N. Goyal et al. "Non Diabetic and Stress Induced Hyperglycemia [SIH] in Orthopaedic Practice: What Do We Know So Far?" *Journal of Clinical and Diagnostic Research* 8, no. 10 (2014): LH01–LH03. https://www.ncbi.nlm.nih.gov/pmc/articles/PMC4253199.

44. "390 Drugs That Can Affect Blood Glucose Levels." Diabetes in Control (2016). http://www.diabetesincontrol.com/drugs-that-can-affect-blood-glucose-levels.

45. "What Medicines Can Make Your Blood Sugar Spike?" WebMD (2017). http://www.webmd.com/diabetes/tc/medicines-that-can-raise-blood-sugar-as-a-side-effect-topic-overview.

46. "Drug-Induced Low Blood Sugar." MedlinePlus (2016). https://medlineplus.gov/ency/article/000310.htm.

47. A. Chiolero et al. "Consequences of Smoking for Body Weight, Body Fat Distribution, and Insulin Resistance." *American Journal of Clinical Nutrition* 87, no. 4 (2008): 801–809. http://ajcn.nutrition.org/content/87/4/801.long.

48. D. Glick. "Women's Monthly Cycle Affects Blood Glucose Control, but Not Consistently." *Diabetes Health*, August 15, 2009. https://www.diabeteshealth.com/womens-monthly-cycle-affects-blood-glucose-control-but-not-consistently.

49. P. Kishore. "Hypoglycemia (Low Blood Sugar)." Merck Manual. http://www.merckmanuals.com/home/hormonal-and-metabolic-disorders/diabetes-mellitus-dm-and-disorders-of-blood-sugar-metabolism/hypoglycemia.

50. K. Chang. "Artificial Sweeteners May Disrupt Body's Blood Sugar Controls." *New York Times*, September 17, 2014. http://well.blogs.nytimes.com/2014/09/17/artificial-sweeteners-may-disrupt-bodys-blood-sugar-controls/?_r=0.

51. "Glycemic Index Testing & Research." The University of Sydney. http://www.glycemicindex.com/testing_research.php.

52. J. W. Conn and L. H. Newburgh. "The Glycemic Response to Isoglucogenic Quantities of Protein and Carbohydrate." *Journal of Clinical Investigation* 15, no. 6 (1936): 665–671. https://www.ncbi.nlm.nih.gov/pmc/articles/PMC424828.

Chapter 7: The Personalized Nutrition Project

1. K. M. Cunningham and N. W. Read. "The Effect of Incorporating Fat into Different Components of a Meal on Gastric Emptying and Postprandial Blood Glucose and Insulin Responses." *British Journal of Nutrition* 61, no. 2 (1989): 285–290. https://www.ncbi.nlm.nih.gov/pubmed/2650735?dopt=Abstract.

2. "What Is Obesity?" *Medical News Today*, January 2016. http://www.medicalnewstoday.com/info/obesity/what-is-bmi.php.

3. L. Karan. "HbA1c Explained." *Type 1 Diabetes Network* (2010). http://t1dn.org.au/our-stuff/all-about-type-1-articles/hba1c-explained.

4. "Tests and Diagnosis." *Mayo Clinic* (2014). http://www.mayoclinic.org/diseases-conditions/diabetes/basics/tests-diagnosis/con-20033091.

5. S. Xiao et al. "A Gut Microbiota–Targeted Dietary Intervention for Amelioration of Chronic Inflammation Underlying Metabolic Syndrome." *FEMS Microbiology Ecology* 87, no. 2 (2014): 357–367. https://www.ncbi.nlm.nih.gov/pubmed/24117923?dopt=Abstract.

6. S. H. Duncan et al. "Reduced Dietary Intake of Carbohydrates by Obese Subjects Results in Decreased Concentrations of Butyrate and Butyrate-Producing Bacteria in Feces." *Applied and Environmental Microbiology* 73, no. 4 (2007): 1073–1078. https://www.ncbi.nlm.nih.gov/pubmed/17189447?dopt=Abstract.

7. V. K. Ridaura et al. "Gut Microbiota from Twins Discordant for Obesity Modulate Metabolism in Mice." *Science* 341, no. 6150 (2013). https://www.ncbi.nlm.nih.gov/pubmed/24009397?dopt=Abstract.

8. P. J. Turnbaugh et al. "An Obesity-Associated Gut Microbiome with Increased Capacity for Energy Harvest." *Nature* 444, no. 7122 (2006): 1027–1031. https://www.ncbi.nlm.nih.gov/pubmed/17183312?dopt=Abstract.

Chapter 8: Testing Your Blood Sugar Responses

1. J. Briffa. "Study Links Blood Sugar Imbalance with Increased Appetite." *Dr. Briffa.* September 3, 2007. http://www.drbriffa.com/2007/09/03/study-links-blood-sugar-imbalance-with-increased-appetite.

2. M. R. Jospe et al. "Adherence to Hunger Training Using Blood Glucose Monitoring: A Feasibility Study." *Nutrition & Metabolism* 12, no. 22 (2015). https://www.ncbi.nlm.nih.gov/pmc/articles/PMC4465140.

Chapter 9: Fine-Tuning Your Personalized Diet

1. P. J. Turnbaugh et al. "The Effect of Diet on the Human Gut Microbiome: A Metagenomic Analysis in Humanized Gnotobiotic Mice." *Science Translational Medicine* 1, no. 6 (2009). https://www.ncbi.nlm.nih.gov/pmc/articles/PMC2894525.

2. "Fat, Sugar Cause Bacterial Changes that May Relate to Loss of Cognitive Function." *Oregon State University*, June 22, 2015. http://oregonstate.edu/ua/ncs/archives/2015/jun/fat-sugar-cause-bacterial-changes-may-relate-loss-cognitive-function.

3. J. L. Sonnenburg and F. Bäckhed. "Diet-Microbiota Interactions as Moderators of Human Metabolism." *Nature* 535, no. 7610 (2016): 56–64. http://www.nature.com/nature/journal/v535/n7610/full/nature18846.html.

4. N. Vordeades et al. "Diet and the Development of the Human Intestinal Microbiome." *Frontiers in Microbiology* 5, no. 494 (2014). https://www.ncbi.nlm.nih.gov/pmc/articles/PMC4170138.

5. S. M. Kuo. "The Interplay between Fiber and the Intestinal Microbiome in the Inflammatory Response." *Advances in Nutrition* 4 (2013): 16–28. http://advances.nutrition.org/content/4/1/16.full.

6. K. H. Courage. "Fiber-Famished Gut Microbes Linked to Poor Health." *Scientific American*, March 23, 2015. https://www.scientificamerican.com/article/fiber-famished-gut-microbes-linked-to-poor-health1.

Chapter 11: The Future of Dieting

1. M. Boyle. "Nestlé Wants to Personalize Your Food." *Bloomberg*, June 26, 2014. https://www.bloomberg.com/news/articles/2014-06-26/star-trek-inspires-nestles-food-nutrition-project.

2. S. C. Mukhopadhyay. "Wearable Sensors for Human Activity Monitoring: A Review." *IEEE Sensors Journal* 15, no. 3 (2015): 1321–1330. http://www.dreamerindia.com/IEEE/IEEE2015/Wearable%20Sensors%20for%20Human%20Activity.pdf.

INDEX

Page numbers of illustrations, charts, and graphs appear in italics.

ABOUT THE AUTHORS

Dr. Eran Segal was born in Tel Aviv, Israel, and received a BSc summa cum laude in computer science from Tel Aviv University in 1998, and a PhD in computer science and genetics from Stanford University in 2004. After holding an independent research position at Rockefeller University, he joined the Weizmann Institute of Science in Israel in 2005, where he is a professor in the Department of Computer Science and Applied Mathematics. Dr. Segal heads a research lab with a multidisciplinary team of computational biologists and experimental scientists in computational and systems biology. His group has extensive experience in machine learning, computational biology, statistical models, and analysis of heterogeneous large-scale data. His research focuses on nutrition, genetics, microbiome, and gene regulation and their effect on health and disease. His aim is to develop personalized nutrition and personalized medicine. The lab website is http://genie.weizmann.ac.il.

Dr. Segal has published more than 120 publications that were cited by more than 25,000 research articles and has received several awards and honors for his work, including the Alon

Foundation award (2006); the EMBO Young Investigator award (2007); the Overton Prize (2007), awarded annually by the International Society for Computational Biology (ISCB) to one scientist for outstanding accomplishments in computational biology; the Levinson Prize in biology (2009); and the Michael Bruno award (2015). The *Scientist* named him a "Scientist to Watch" (2009), and Sonima elected him as one of fifty innovators. In 2012, he was elected as a member of the Young Israel Academy of Science, and in 2015, he was elected as an EMBO member.

Dr. Segal is married to Keren and lives in Ramat Hasharon, Israel, with his three children, Shira, Yoav, and Tamar; their cat Blue; and their dog Snow. He is an avid long-distance runner who has completed ten full marathons.

DR. ERAN ELINAV was born in Jerusalem and completed his medical doctor's (MD) degree at the Hebrew University of Jerusalem summa cum laude in 2000, followed by a clinical internship, residency in internal medicine, and a clinical and research position at the Tel Aviv Medical Center Gastroenterology Institute. In 2009, he received a PhD in immunology from the Weizmann Institute of Science, followed by a postdoctoral fellowship at Yale University School of Medicine. Dr. Elinav is a professor heading a multidisciplinary research group of more than thirty immunologists, microbiologists, metabolic experts, and computational biologists at the Department of Immunology, Weizmann Institute of Science. His lab focuses on deciphering the molecular basis of host-microbiome interactions and their effects on health and disease, with a goal of personalizing medicine and nutrition. The Elinav lab employs diverse, state-of-the-art experimental, genomic, and computational methods to study the involvement of gut microbes in diverse multifactorial diseases, including obesity and its metabolic complications, inflammatory and autoimmune disorders, neurodegenerative disease and cancer, with an aim to develop microbiome-targeting personalized treatment modalities for these disorders. His lab website is http://www.weizmann.ac.il/immunology/elinav.

Dr. Elinav has published more than 120 publications in leading peer-reviewed journals and has received several awards for his discoveries, including the Claire and Emmanuel G. Rosenblatt award from the American Physicians for Medicine (2011); the Alon Foundation award (2013); the 2015 Rappaport Prize for biomedical research, awarded annually to a single scientist for breakthrough biomedical discoveries; the 2016 Lindner award; Israeli Society of Endocrinology's highest prize; and the 2016 Levinson award for basic science research (2016). Dr. Elinav is also a senior fellow at the Canadian Institute for Advanced Research (CIFAR), an elected member of the European Molecular Biology Association (EMBO), and is an international scholar at the Howard Hughes Medical Institute (HHMI).

Dr. Elinav is married to Hila and lives in Mazkeret Batya, Israel, with his three children, Shira, Omri, and Inbal, and their dog Herzl. In his spare time, he likes to mountain trek and ski.